DAMAC

In 1951, when Jean ... tuberculosis, she was only thirteen years old. At a time when for most girls the possibilities of life are opening up, Jean was separated from her friends, taken from her home and confined in a sanatorium. Here, in spite of new so-called wonder drugs and innovative treatment techniques, the battle against TB was often lost. Many of the friendships Jean made were to end in death, and it was to be four years before her own life-saving operation and her return home.

Jean believes she learned more from her time in Law Hospital than she has ever learned since. Now, looking back over those years in Law Hospital, she explains how in spite of everything she will always be grateful to the staff and fellow patients who taught her so much.

DAMAGED BLOOMS

Jean Anderson

ARTHUR H. STOCKWELL LTD
Torrs Park, Ilfracombe, Devon, EX34 8BA
Established 1898
www.ahstockwell.co.uk

First published in Great Britain, 2019

British Library Cataloguing-in-Publication Data.
A catalogue record for this book is available from the British Library.

ISBN 978-0-7223-4873-4
Printed in Great Britain by
Arthur H. Stockwell Ltd
Torrs Park Ilfracombe
Devon EX34 8BA

CONTENTS

Introduction		7
Part 1	Law Hospital	19
Chapter 1	Admitted to the Sanatorium	21
Chapter 2	Visiting Time and Letters from Home	31
Chapter 3	Ward 28	34
Chapter 4	Results Days	45
Chapter 5	Ina	59
Chapter 6	Flora	66
Chapter 7	Pen Pals	74
Chapter 8	Goodbyes	86
Chapter 9	The Convalescent Ward	97
Chapter 10	Mrs God Bless You and Other Good Souls	103
Part 2	Hairmyers Hospital	109
Chapter 1	New Friends	111
Chapter 2	A Life-Saving Operation	129

INTRODUCTION

My best pal, Isa Biggam, and I were sitting on the backs of the fireside chairs, our feet on the squeaky Rexine seats. We were singing 'Red Sails in the Sunset' to one another. It was our favourite song of the moment. Wee Johnnie was trying to get round the room without touching the floor – he had got as far as the sideboard and was stretching his wee chubby pork-link leg for the window ledge. My other young brother, Ross, and I had taught him this game. It kept him out of the road for hours on end.

The summons we had been waiting for came from the next room – a rap on the wall that told us Daddy wanted his ten-o'clock tea. We slid down from the chairs, feeling our skin pull as if a large Elastoplast was being pulled off our bare thighs. It was a pain we liked. We liked everything about Saturday mornings. Every week was the same. Our mammy took the two older brothers, Eddie and Robert, with her to the Co-op to help carry the week's messages; my two big sisters, Margaret and Anna, either worked or went up the town; Ross went off on a wee boy's mysterious mission with his pal McGinn; and Isa came to help me to look after wee Johnnie and see that Daddy got his racing paper and wasn't disturbed in his long lie-in.

As soon as he knocked on the wall we knew what to do.

"You put the kettle on and I'll see if he wants me to go for cakes," I told Isa, who was already lighting the gas on the cooker.

This was the best part of the Saturday ritual. He would tell one of us to go and get cakes for a 'wee fly cup'. Wee Johnnie would get a barley-sugar stick or a lolly stuck in his hand and we would sit on the bed, eating cakes, drinking tea and giggling at Daddy's patter. Only one thing had been spoiling Saturdays lately – my stupid cough.

"Take some of that bronchial stuff your mother got for me," Daddy said as I took the tea in. "You know how to make it up, don't you?"

I did, but I also knew it didn't help. Nothing did.

"What did that doctor say about it last week anyway? You would think you smoked forty Woodbines a day to hear you."

This made Isa and me giggle so much that we didn't hear the rattle on the metal knocker of the front door at first. We called it the front door, although it was the middle door on the second-floor landing of a three-storey tenement. It was our front door.

Isa and I went to open it together. We always acted together. It was a man! Enough to make us turn red and cross our legs in excitement. He was young – obviously a toff, because he was wearing a hat and carrying a wee case of some sort (I should have recognised him, as he was the locum from the doctors' surgery, but I was too drowning in shyness to do so).

"Is your mother or father in?" he asked, looking almost as flustered as us.

"My father's in, but he's in bed," I answered, kicking Isa for laughing at my 'pan-loaf' voice.

Before we knew it he was standing in the long lobby that led from the front door to the rest of the house. Daddy's bedroom was the very last one of the three, next to the living-room door.

"Which is your father's room?" he asked, and I pointed it out.

We followed him to the bedroom door – sure that he was a burglar or a murderer – but he shut it in our faces as he entered, having given a loud, angry knock.

"Who the hell are you?"

We settled down to listen at the door as we heard Daddy's growl, but there was a sudden thump from the living room and a cry that told us that wee Johnnie still couldn't reach the window sill from the sideboard without touching the floor and we had to go and pacify him.

* * * * *

"I'm your daughter's doctor."

Ned drew angrily on his cigarette as he glared at what seemed to him to be no more than a frightened boy in a man's suit, weighed down on one side by an oversized doctor's bag. He was not happy at his long lie-in being interrupted. 'Bloody insurance man!' was his first thought until he noticed the bag and heard the lad's answer to his question.

"Keep calm, Mr Wales," he said in a firm voice, which did not go with his young, nervous face." I've come to talk to you on a very important matter concerning your daughter Jean's health. I'm afraid she's a very sick wee girl."

Ned thought right away about the cough. He had been thinking about it a lot recently. It brought back memories – memories he did not want to let in. He remembered a cousin and then his own sister, wasting away to death in their early teens, and the tearing coughs they had had. But that was before the war – people were healthier now. It couldn't be anything like that with their Jean. Hadn't Peggy had her at the Doctor's just last Friday? She'd had an X-ray. That would be it. The boy had got the result of it and had come to let them know and probably brought a prescription – that was really decent of him. About time they were doing something! That cough had been going on for months now and Peggy said she was off her food. The Doctor had told her it was probably her age. She was outgrowing her strength. It would right itself in time.

"I'm sorry to tell you, Mr Wales, your daughter has contracted tuberculosis. It's in both lungs."

Ned noticed the young man's Adam's apple disappear under his frayed collar for moment, before jumping out like a bubble in porridge.

"It's really far advanced – how on earth did she get into

this state before anything was done about it? Surely you must have noticed she was ill?"

"I did notice she had a bit of a cough," Ned answered. He was beginning to feel black burning shame – that he was being accused of neglecting his daughter by this young lad. "But she's always full o' life and her mother's had her to the Doctor's umpteen times about the cough – was it not you? – and she was told it was down to her age, or she was just trying to get time off school. Ach, to be honest, son, I don't often see the wee lassie. Is she really that bad?"

The words he had heard his aunts and his granny saying in whispers all those years ago, when his cousin and then his sister had died, kept forcing their way into his mind – 'galloping consumption'. That had been the name given to TB then. As a wee boy the words had formed themselves into an image of a vicious, black, glistening horse, teeth dripping with the blood of its victims as it galloped through his nightmares.

But that had been years ago. There would be medicines now to cure it.

"I'm sorry," the Doctor answered. "It really is bad. I wish she had been X-rayed sooner, but I didn't see your daughter until this morning. I'm only a locum, standing in for her regular doctor. When I saw the results of the X-ray this morning I came right here. I'm not going to raise your hopes, Mr Wales, but there are drugs which are supposed to be working wonders. Let's hope they do it it for Jean. He walked towards the door, turning a contemptuous glare on Ned. "See that she has a warm bath and get her into bed right away. Try to keep things quiet for her and don't let her mix with other children if possible. I'll be back on Monday with her first dose of drugs, and I'll put her name on the waiting list for a bed in a sanatorium." His voice was more sad than angry. "I hope we've caught her in time."

As Dr Murdo Nicolson hurried out of the housing-scheme tenement, longing for his parents' red-roofed bungalow in Newton Mearns, he cursed the mistakes and oversights made by the sick old doctor he was replacing. He cursed the man to whom he had just been speaking – lying there, surrounded by racing papers and fags, having a lie-in while his daughter was dying before his eyes.

"Scum of the earth," he judged from his ivory tower of middle-class superiority.

Ned got up and got dressed as soon as the door closed. What was the best way to tackle the things he had to do? What could he say to his daughter? He only knew her as the skinny, giggly young thing who brought his Saturday-morning tea and sat at the living-room table doing homework most nights. He should have known from that that she was not using the cough to get time off school, as that fool of a doctor had said. At least this young lad seemed to know what he was doing.

Jesus Christ! Just the other night he had refused to let her leave the table at teatime because she hadn't finished her egg and chips, which they had heard her spewing up in the bathroom as soon as he had made her force it down.

He blamed Peggy.

* * * * *

Of all the things that happened in my life, before and after that day, nothing was as permanent and left as vivid a memory as the scene that took place between me and Daddy after the Doctor left that morning. It came back to me during moments of triumph, sadness and love. Whether I was alone or in a crowd, it made me into that little girl of thirteen again, trying to take in and understand those strange new feelings that were like a suit of ill-fitting clothes – yet wonderful.

Daddy came out of the bedroom and stood looking at Isa and me, sitting at opposite ends of the horsehair sofa. We didn't know whether to ask about the visitor or not. Daddy could be funny sometimes. It was a bit like sitting outside the headmaster's door, waiting for judgment to be pronounced for some serious crime – like not wearing a school tie.

"You're like two bookends sitting there," he said, and we giggled in relief and made faces at one another.

He stood, for what seemed ages, just looking at us, making our nerves start up again. He wasn't even smoking.

"Your wee pal's got to go home now," he said at last. "That was the Doctor. He says you should be in bed. Nothing to worry about – just that you should get some rest." Turning to Isa: "Off you go, hen. You can come back and see Jean later, when she's better."

Isa grabbed her coat and left, looking miserable.

I had never been alone with him before. Wee Johnnie was there, but he was sound asleep.

What I remember most is not that he told me I was very ill and would be going into hospital. I had had a good idea for a long time that there was something bad about the cough, and the fact that I never wanted to eat, and going into hospital quite appealed to me. I saw myself as one of the heroines in the hospital romances that Isa and I loved. It was the way he told me.

He held my hand.

Nobody had ever done that before. We were a family who did not touch one another in affection. We did not kiss and cuddle – even on birthdays. We felt shame for and ridiculed any show of physical affection in others. It was sissy.

The dour Scot is not a creation of fiction. He learns to be that way at his mother's knee – at arm's length, of course.

He spoke to me in a calm, serious voice that made my teeth chatter, telling me that I had to have a nice warm bath and get into bed. "Rest is all you need," he said, and squeezed my hand.

I felt like crying or shouting aloud and throwing myself on to his lap. I wanted to lose myself in him. It was as if until then I, Jean Wales, had never been a real, touchable person. It was as if he had discovered who I was and let me into a secret that only he and I knew.

The instructions from the Doctor that I should have a warm bath straight away showed the great social divide between him and most of his patients. He could draw himself a warm bath any time he liked; but for me to be able to have such a thing, the living-room fire had to be 'backed up' with coal for hours before the water would be hot enough for even one bath, and Isa and

I had almost let it go out that morning – we had been too busy singing. It would be hours before the shovelfuls Daddy heaped on it would give birth to any hot water.

"I'll boil the kettle and you can give yourself a good wash in the big sink," he said as he unfolded the bed-chair in the living room. He said the Doctor thought it would be better if I did not sleep with my sisters until I was better.

I cared about nothing. I was so high with happiness.

"Where's your nightie or pyjamas?"

Suddenly there was embarrassment between us. I slept in my knickers and vest. The only person I knew who owned pyjamas was wee Johnnie. I didn't answer, feeling that there was something shameful in not having pyjamas. My sisters didn't have them either. They slept in their underskirts. Were we the only family so depraved?

"Never mind," he winked. "I'll give you one of my old army shirts. That'll keep you warm until your mammy gets you pyjamas. You'll need them for going into hospital. You'll need a lot of things."

I shot up to the ceiling again. Life seemed good to me.

"The Doctor says you have to eat something," he said quietly as I got under the old grey army blanket after my wash at the kitchen sink.

We were short of sheets – it was only when I got into hospital that I realised that people slept with a sheet on top as well as under. We always had plenty of blankets. Daddy acquired them from the barracks at Maryhill, where he had worked in the stores before he was finally demobbed.

Nothing has ever felt so comforting since as the rough, jaggy blanket did against my cold body that day.

* * * * *

'Jesus Christ, no wonder that young fella was mad,' Ned thought as he made tea in the kitchen (he had even forgotten about putting on a bet that day). 'She looks like a bloody Belsen horror.' He had peeked in as she stood at the sink, stripped to her vest and knickers, and noticed the bones sticking out of her back and shoulders and her stick-insect legs. 'If I'd been told, it wouldna have gone as far as this. He's right – she's been neglected.'

He heard Peggy's key in the door and his two sons' voices as they returned with the messages. He stepped out of the kitchen and barred their way into the living room.

"You two, go out and play for an hour," he told the boys roughly. "I need to talk to your mother."

They turned to go without question and he wondered, not for the first time, why they seemed to be afraid of him.

"Why did you not tell me how ill that wee lassie is?" he accused, giving her no time to put down her shopping bag or get her breath. "I've had a doctor in here this morning, practically accusing me of neglect, and when I see the state of her I don't blame him. What the hell have you been playin' at? She could die."

"Is it Jean?" she asked, knowing it was a senseless question. "What's wrong? I told you she wasnae well. I've had her at the Doctor dozens of times. I took her for an X-ray last week – you know that. Where is she?"

She made for the door of the middle bedroom, where the girls normally slept, but he grabbed her arm.

"She's in the living room. It's TB. She's not to sleep with her sisters. He's going to try to get her into a hospital. I'm going for a pint. Make sure she gets something decent to eat. She's like something out o' a concentration camp."

With that he grabbed his coat from the rack in the lobby and walked out.

Peggy poured herself a cup of tea and stood staring out of the kitchenette window, where the Harland and Wolff building could be seen beyond the railway goods yard, over the wall from the back court with the crumbling air-raid shelter, still standing five years after the war. She didn't see any of them. Her eyes were unfocused. The unfairness and cruelty of what Ned had said about her neglecting Jean hurt her physically. Her throat constricted like a clenched fist and she couldn't swallow the tears that she despised herself for shedding.

'He's right,' she thought miserably. She should have made that old doctor do something sooner. She had taken his word that the lassie was all right. Now she was going to die. TB – you never heard of anyone getting better from that. She had never questioned the rightness of what Ned said – never since the first time he had taken her to the park and had her virginity, when she was sixteen.

Yet she felt that this man who had come back from the war was not that Ned. He had made her laugh and proudly took his weans out in the pram – a new baby every two years, and left her with six to bring up when he was called into the army. She supposed that the war had changed a lot of men, but did they all despise their wives and families as much as he did? Still, things had seemed to be better since they moved back to Glasgow. The news about Jean, their youngest daughter, had put paid to that, and she felt sometimes that he hated all of them.

* * * * *

If I hadn't felt so bad, I would have enjoyed lying there like the Lady of the Camellias (the Greta Garbo film had been in the local picture house two weeks ago and Isa and I had revelled in the romance of the beautiful dying heroine); but as it was I cowered under the blankets, wishing it was night-time and I would be left alone. Everybody seemed embarrassed more than anything. They carried on with their usual pastimes as if I had somehow disappeared. They were the way people are sometimes with blind people or those in wheelchairs. They never looked in my direction or spoke to me. The connection between us had been broken.

They all carried on with what they were doing when they heard Daddy's key in the door, but there was a quietness that had not been there before. They were waiting to behave the way his mood dictated. If he was in a good mood, they could relax and he would maybe join in some of their games or kid Annie about the home perm she was giving herself. If he was in a bad mood, glaring and bristling at them, they would find excuses to leave the room – sometimes even going to bed without having to be told.

He was in a good mood.

Everyone – apart from me – laughed with relief as he took packets of sweets from every pocket and threw them on the ironing board in front of Mammy, who blushed and let on she was annoyed. (This was more like the Ned she had known before the war.) She smiled as he threw each of them a packet – Dolly Mixtures for wee Johnnie, Sharps caramels for the boys, and Paradise Fruits for Mammy, Anna and Margaret – nothing for me.

Anna held out her packet to me, but he laughed and said, "You eat them yourself, hen. I've brought something special for my wee sick girl."

And the others watched – green to the gills as he produced a golden chocolate box tied with a red ribbon.

"You've to eat every one yourself. We need to get you fattened up – that's what the Doctor said."

He ruffled my hair and sat on the bed-chair beside me. It was too much – I burst into shameful tears.

"What are ye greetin' for?" Ross said. "I wish I could get a box of chocolates all to myself. You're lucky."

I wiped my face on the blanket, suddenly happily aware of my new position as the centre of attention in the family. In the coming days Daddy made sure that everyone knew that I was the most important person in the household and they must behave accordingly.

Everybody reacted differently: Margaret continued to ignore me as a lower form of life; Anna, good-natured Anna, who took everything in her stride, took it hardest. We had slept in the same bed and we had always had great laughs, her telling me about the dancing, singing the latest songs to me and making me giggle, and me telling her about what my pal Isa and I got up to. She was my hero.

The older boys, Eddie and Robert, looked at me with new interest for a day or two and then went back to ignoring me; Ross and Johnnie were jealous of the treats I got, Ross particularly envious that I didn't have to go to school, which he hated and dodged out of when he could. Still, I thought he was quite sad, but could never say it.

* * * * *

Ned felt hopeful about his life that night as he sat on the wee sick girl's bed and talked to the rest of his family. Maybe they were not such a useless lot as he had come to think. That was Peggy's fault. She had turned the boys into sissies who resented him. The lasses were fine, apart from Margaret taking up with a Catholic. He blamed Peggy for that too.

Peggy felt good too – the happiest she'd felt for months. It was great that he was chatting away to her and the weans, telling the older ones that they must visit their sister when she went into the hospital, so that she would not be lonely.

* * * * *

"That was the first time you had really talked to us all like that. You only ever spoke to the boys to check them," I told him when I was back home after the years in the hospital.

"None of you ever spoke to me," he answered. "I'd just lived for being back wi' my family. I wanted to help you all get on – do the things I'd never had the chance to do, get an education and decent jobs – but none of you ever spoke to me unless I spoke first. Well, you did sometimes. You were different from the rest of them. I suppose that's why I paid more attention to you than the rest. You had more of a personality and I used to see my sister Nancy in you." He laughed. "You were always reading and your mother got mad at you. She was always saying you were lazy and never did a hand's turn in the house. I remember you used to sit opposite me, by the fireside, not caring if the world fell about your ears, with your wee snottery nose stuck in a book and your knees up to your chest – showing your navy-blue knickers to the world. I noticed there was a big hole in them and gave

Anna money to buy you new ones. Your mother never seemed to bother."

I felt a bit guilty about not defending the rest of the family to him, but my pleasure at knowing he had noticed me – even if it was embarrassing – defeated my better feelings.

It was only two weeks after that Saturday morning – no, two weeks and two days, because it was on a Monday – that they came for me.

Daddy had taken a day off work and made Mammy's life a misery of nagging and finding fault while they waited for the ambulance that was to take me to a sanatorium somewhere in Lanarkshire. I felt too ill to fully enjoy the drama of being carried out through the neighbour-lined close on a stretcher, covered to my chin in a bright-red blanket. The thought came to me that hospital blankets must be red so as not to show up the blood.

Mammy came into the ambulance with me – I had never seen her face so white and unhappy – and told me not to worry, that I would soon be better and that she would come to visit me on Wednesday, which was the first visiting day. Daddy stood at the close, smoking and ignoring the sympathetic clucking of the women, who had left their fireplaces and kitchens at the first sign of an ambulance in the street.

"Poor wee soul," our fat downstairs neighbour said, shaking her head in its metal curlers and wiping a dry tear from her eye.

Ross and I were convinced that the curlers must be joined to her head as she was never seen without them.

I felt really sad for the wee girl being taken to some far-off sanatorium, away from all she loved and perhaps never coming back (my thoughts were often in the language of the *Red Star Weekly*) or, failing that, meeting a smashing-looking doctor who would save her life, marry her and take her to live in Milngavie, or somewhere posh like that. I had just been reading a Nurse Barton book with a plot just like that, but if I had known that my stay in hospital would be a lot different from my romantic ideas, and take nearly four years out of my life, I would have been off that stretcher and away.

Part 1

LAW HOSPITAL

CHAPTER 1

ADMITTED TO THE SANATORIUM

Law Hospital, situated on the edge of a small Lanarkshire village, overlooked by a black, menacing coal bing, which was being softened in its outline by the brave growth of young grass on its slopes, had been used partly as a military hospital during the war – well, the part in which I was to spend four years of my life, that is. It had been turned into a sanatorium for TB cases, of which I was one.

It was 1951, and the life-saving drugs that were eventually to defeat the disease were still in the experimental stage. TB was still a plague in Glasgow, as it was throughout Britain. Many cases were being detected in the fairly early stages because of the Mass Radiography Programme, which had been put into operation by a forward-thinking health board. With the introduction of the new drugs, pioneering surgery and other treatments, the scourge was soon to be as good as wiped out, so that now few people remember its devastating effects on rich and poor alike.

I was thirteen years old when I was diagnosed with what the older people called 'galloping consumption'. I had been fighting a losing battle against a scary hacking cough, which made me sound about ninety years old. A teacher had mislaid the consent forms of our class, so I missed out on being X-rayed and we had a family doctor who was overworked and, in any case, believed that all adolescent girls were 'too full of imagination for their own good'.

His advice – accompanied by a bottle of iron tonic – was

"Make sure she eats her food and takes plenty of outdoor exercise. There's nothing wrong with her. It's just her age."

Probably the best piece of luck I ever had in my life was when this 'caring individual' was off on holiday and a young locum was brought in. One of my teachers had sent me home early with a note advising my mother to 'Take Jean to her doctor. She fell asleep in class today and is not at all well.'

My mother was totally humiliated, feeling that she probably seemed like a neglectful mother – but at that time what the Doctor said was gospel and she was following his advice.

I suppose that I was beginning to realise that something was really wrong with me. I had been quite enjoying the attention I got, being sent out of class to get a drink of water when my cough was driving everyone mad and being allowed to sit out of PT lessons by a woman who normally seemed to be trying to kill us all by the severity of the exercises she made us perform – even on 'bad days', as we referred to our menstruation cycle. It was becoming more and more difficult to make my body drag itself to the school bus and I could not put food in my mouth without being sick. If this was 'imagination' I wanted rid of it – quickly.

I coughed the whole time we sat in the musty waiting room, getting tuts of sympathy and head-shakings from the other patients. The thought of the crabbit old GP and what he would say to us this time was making me feel guilty for daring to come back to him after the 'imagination' remark, and my mother, Peggy, was getting more and more flushed with embarrassment.

"I don't know what people must have thought – her coughing like that!" she said in affronted tones as she described the scene later on to my father, Ned.

At first I thought there must be some mistake, because, instead of the usual old grump, there was a lad who looked about the age of the 'big boys' at my school – the smart ones who were 'staying on' in preparation for going to university – who were remote godlike figures to be worshipped from afar by wee girls like me and my pals.

"Hello," he said, offering his hand to be shaken. "I'm Dr Nicolson – Dr Wyman is away for a while. Sit down and tell me how I can help." And, turning to me: "Who is this young lady?"

I don't know whose blush was more intense – Mum's or mine. We felt totally nonplussed by the fact that anyone so young could be a doctor. However, his genuine interest in my problems was obvious from the intent way he listened and the way he never took his eyes off me, and soon Mum was telling him the history of my cough and how it was 'pulling me down'. She even felt confident enough to tell him that she had been unhappy with Dr Wyman's diagnosis – although she stammered a bit over telling him this.

I studied him while he was sounding my chest: he was very slim (probably that made him look even younger than he was) and fair-skinned, yet his hair and eyes were dark and I could see that there was a slight shadow on his sharp chin, showing that he did have to shave – but so did a lot of the 'big boys'. I noticed the frown that was deepening on his brow as he listened through his stethoscope, and I stopped being embarrassed about my scrawny little breasts: what on earth was he hearing to worry him so?

"I want you to take your daughter for a chest X-ray as soon as I can arrange it," he said, turning from me to the desk and beginning to scribble on a card. "I'll make an appointment at Florence Street Clinic for tomorrow morning. Take this card with you." He shook his head at me, the way some teachers did when I didn't know the answer to a question. "We want to get you better as soon as we can, young lady. You won't want to miss too much school, eh?"

He laughed, but I could see that he was just trying to make me feel all right – and in a way he did, but not because of his 'joke'; the very fact of having a young, good-looking doctor attending to me was going to give me enough material to pin back my pals' ears for quite a time.

Florence Street was an experience I never forgot. It was packed with people waiting for chest X-rays. The procedure was that you gave your appointment card to a sour-faced receptionist, who said, "Sit in room four 'til your name's called," without giving you the courtesy of a glance.

Room four was painted predominately bottle green with dreary brown trimmings. All round the wall were hard wooden chairs – of the kind that fold up – mostly occupied by people who looked as if they were waiting for judgement day (I suppose they were in a way). Every few minutes one or more of them would go out of the room and come back wafting the smell of nicotine. At other times a trim little nurse came to the door, called a name and escorted the named person from the room. The coughing was the worst thing about the room: hacking dry coughs, wet sputum-filled coughs, high-pitched coughs, deep chesty coughs, and some that included all varieties. Some spat into hankies; others gulped and swallowed back the poison their lungs were trying to eject – too embarrassed to spit. I was sure I had been sent to the wrong room. My pathetic little cough was a mouse's squeak compared to these.

"Is it the wee lassie you're here wi'?" a yellow-faced woman sitting beside Mum asked, shaking her head sadly when told I was the patient. "Well," she went on, "at least she'll be able to get the new wonder drug that's out. Did ye read about it in the *Sunday Mail*? It's a few years too late for me, ah think, eh?" Her laugh brought on a scary fit of coughing and she studied the contents of her hankie with a philosophical shake of her head. "Ah'll away for a smoke before they shout my name. It'll no be long now, pet," she added, patting my shoulder as she lurched out, still hacking and clutching her hankie to her mouth.

After that I got a lot of sympathetic looks (which with the disdain of an adolescent I treated with contempt). I found these people disgusting and was sure that, whatever was wrong with me, it was not the same as what they had.

But it was.

On the Saturday morning, just over a week after my appointment at Florence Street, Dr Nicolson (I recognised him now) arrived at our door with the news which mapped the route of the rest of my life and made changes for the whole family.

My best pal and I were watching my wee brother while Mum was shopping and the rest of the siblings were on their various missions of Saturday freedom. Dad was having a long lie-in, studying 'the horses' and calling frequently for cups of tea, which it was my job to make. The loud rattle on the door knocker made Isa and me jump out of our skins and hug one another – we had just finished reading 'The Monkey's Paw' together and Dad shouted to us to open the door before he had to get up and do it himself.

"Hello, Jean," my hero said, blushing as redly as me. "Are your parents in? I need to speak to them."

I stood with my mouth hanging open glaikitly and it was Isa who answered him: "Her mum's away for the messages and her daddy's in bed," she said, eyes glittering with excitement.

"Who is it?" my father shouted from the bedroom.

"It's the Doctor," I found my voice to answer back.

"Well, bring him in here and don't have him standing at the door," the angry voice growled back.

The Doctor passed us and followed the direction of the voice into Dad's room.

"Good morning, Mr Wales. Sorry to disturb you. . . ."

And that was all we heard before he closed the door.

They were in there for ages and we could hear their voices, but not what they were saying. When the door finally opened Dad came out along with the Doctor. He had put on his khaki trousers and a sweater and shook hands as he showed him out.

"Thanks for coming to tell us right away," he said. "It was good of you. We'll see you on Monday, then." His voice turned hoarse. "Thanks again, son."

That morning was the finish of one stage of my life and the beginning of another – one in which I would become part of a separate culture, because that was what life in the sanatorium was. The women there were cut off from their children, lovers and husbands (apart from hour-long visits three times a week, which did not always happen for all the patients), and they had replaced their outside lives with habits, language and rituals to suit the insular lifestyle they were forced to lead, in the shadow of the coal bing.

Before I got a bed in Law Hospital, I felt that I was already separated from what had been my normal 'little girl' existence. Dad had gently told Isa that she must go home as I had to rest in bed, on the Doctor's instructions, and that she was not to come and visit me until I was better. What I did not know, until years later, when I had proved his predictions wrong, was that poor young Dr Nicolson had had to tell Dad that the odds against my surviving were like those of an outsider winning the Grand National.

So I had 'lost' my pal. The next to go were my two young brothers. Despite staying in the same overcrowded house, the instructions from the 'green lady' (the district nurse) were that they should be kept away from me as much as possible.

"I know whole families who have the disease because it is so contagious, so you must be very careful," she told Mum. "At least it will only be for a few weeks. Dr Nicolson thinks he can get her a bed in Law Hospital, near Carluke. I hope he's right."

The rest of the family agreed that they were not going to treat me 'like a leper', but, looking back, I think that they were really scared of catching 'it'. All of them got the all-clear when they were X-rayed, so we were not going to be like one of those 'whole families' of the green lady's experience. Both she and my doctor hero visited me every day, so obviously the risk meant nothing to them.

Easter Monday was the day on which the ambulance arrived at the close to take me away. He told me as he saw me into the ambulance that a week from then he had to report for his stint of national service, and Nurse Wright (the green lady) told me that she was emigrating to Canada on that same day. I felt that there was some kind of omen in this news, but I couldn't think whether it was bad or good. All three of us were ending one life and beginning another, although they did not believe in my beginning.

The ambulance had attracted a curious crowd of neighbours and passers-by and the actress in me enjoyed being centre stage – peering over the bright-red hospital blanket and trying to look like Greta Garbo in *Camille*, which Isa and I had seen in a cinema which showed 'classic films'. I even tried a pathetic little cough as I was lifted into my chariot, calling forth utterances of "Poor wee soul" and "Keep your pecker up, hen."

The doors shut and my life was never the same again, although I realise I am lucky to have a life, unlike many of the women I was to meet in Law Hospital.

Before we even reached the hospital I met two of my fellow patients. The driver stopped to pick them up. One was a stretcher case, like me; the other walked on under her own steam.

"Right, girls," the driver said in the cheerful, slightly embarrassed tone I was soon to become used to from many different voices, "introduce yourselves. You're lucky to have pals from the same area. They come from all over to Law."

His mate tucked a blanket round the woman who had walked on and went to sit in front, leaving the three of us in bashful silence.

The woman spoke first: "I'm Jenny Christie," she said in the voice of a sixty-a-day ciggie lover, which came oddly from her ladylike frame.

She was dressed in the kind of expensive tailored suit that I had only ever seen before on schoolteachers or at the pictures. In fact there was a touch of Bette Davis in her appearance and manner, although the thick heavy-framed glasses she wore made her face a bit toad-like to my cruel eyes.

"The driver's right," she went on: "it'll be nice to already know someone when we arrive – eh?"

"I'm Teresa Gray," the figure on the other stretcher said, her voice muffled by the blanket, which seemed on the point of smothering her. "I've never been in hospital before, have you? They say these places are awful. They make you sleep outside—"

Jenny hushed her before she could say more: "Wheesht! You'll frighten the wee lassie," she said, and then, leaning over me kindly: "What's your name, pet?"

Despite the glasses and the smell of tobacco, I liked her. I wasn't sure about the other one, particularly when a hand topped with long dirty nails emerged from her blanket and she began clawing at her dirty-looking mop of black greasy hair. She looked like the kind of girl we had always been told not to play with.

"You never know what you might catch," Mum told us.

Poor Teresa; poor Jenny! Teresa was put into a bed directly opposite mine in the long thirty-bed ward; Jenny was led, by a plump cheerful nurse with incredibly pale eyelashes, to a bed at the far end from us. We were 'bed-patients'; she was an 'up-patient' – able to walk around.

The screens were put around our beds and we were subject to rituals which reminded me of the school nurse's visits – apart from the bed bath, which made me blush for hours after it.

The ward sister was examining my head, like a monkey grooming its partner, when the fair nurse – Nurse McKinnon – put her head round the end of the screen and said, "Excuse me, Sister, could you come and look at this?"

Sister made the annoyed tutting sound which I came to know very well in the years to come and followed her from behind the screen, leaving me with a towel around my shoulders, hair parted in the middle and taking in the familiar smell of 'nit ointment' from a bowl on the tray by my bed. I wished I was home.

My curiosity about why she had been called away was soon to be satisfied.

"You're no cutting my hair off, you wicked auld bitch. Get off me!" The wail coming from outside the screen made me shiver with fear. I recognised Teresa's voice.

Oh, Mammy, Daddy! Would I be next? I wondered if I would have the strength to get out of bed and run away – knowing full well I was trapped in this awful place.

Nurse McKinnon suddenly put her lovely sweet face round the screens and said, "Right now, that's you all nice and clean. We'll get you settled for your lunch, will we?"

As the screens were moved from around my bed I saw another nurse wheeling a glass-shelved trolley, containing sinister covered trays and bowls, behind the screens surrounding poor Teresa, who was now howling like a teething baby.

I really didn't want to look when the screens opposite were finally removed after breakfast the next morning, but I was thirteen years old and Teresa's bed was directly in my line of sight. I did manage not to laugh or gasp in horror – to my credit.

The up-patients hurried as quickly as they could past her bed – and no wonder! Her head was covered with a turban, like the ones I had seen factory girls wearing, in a dark-blue colour which emphasised the yellowness of her compexion and her eyes were half closed from crying – I had heard the night nurse trying to hush her on her rounds, but she had gone on sobbing and moaning until the early hours. She was quiet now, propped up, staring straight ahead, chewing at the inside of her mouth, but at least quiet – until Sister entered the ward with her medicine trolley. It made quite a cheerful tinkling sound and she smiled as if she was bringing goodies to us instead of vile-tasting medicines and agonising injections for poor, tender, pincushion bums.

"Don't you come near me, ye fuckin' auld witch," Teresa shouted, before going into a fit of 'dirty' coughing.

"Now now, Mrs Gray. Control yourself. You mustn't shout – it's bad for you – and there's no need to use that kind of language to Sister." This from the young nurse waiting to pass the various concoctions from Sister to patient.

Sister said nothing, but her jowls, covered with white down, shook and her plump cheeks almost burst they turned so red. She handed Teresa's medicine to the Nurse and hurried on to the next bed, looking like a violated old maid – which in a way she was. At the age of around forty, she was unmarried and truly dedicated to the nursing profession, yet she never unbent to the extent of having a joke with the patients or her staff. Still, I soon had reason to know how truly kind and dedicated she was, although she felt it nearly impossible to relax her professional starchiness.

As the days went by, Teresa continued to glare at everyone and refuse to let anyone remove her turban, even when they gave her a bed bath. It was one of the doctors in charge of the TB ward – Dr Morton – who finally ended the stand-off, by whipping it off as she went on her rounds. Teresa gave one mournful wail and pulled the blankets over her head, but not before her hedgehog haircut had been seen by all of the patients at 'our' end of the ward.

In my ignorance I asked one of the orderlies why Sister had cut poor Teresa's hair.

"She was crawling wi' nits, that's why" was her answer, voiced with quite a measure of spite. "Sister has to think of the other patients, ye know – these things spread. There's nae excuse for a grown woman havin' a dirty head."

Teresa soon got over her unhappy beginning in the ward and became quite friendly, waving over to me and asking how I was getting on. She was blooming. Getting good regular meals and treatment with the new 'wonder drugs' was having an amazing effect on her, and soon she was allowed up to the bathroom to get washed. I felt a bit jealous because she was leaving me behind. I did not seem to be responding to the drugs as well as the doctors had hoped.

My other fellow passenger in the ambulance – Jenny – was a regular visitor to my bedside, bringing me magazines and sweets. She always looked really ill, with her bent back and sunken cheeks, yet her grooming was immaculate. Even in her chenille dressing gown, in the mornings, she always looked as if she was prepared for visitors (who never came), with her pretty blouses, perfect make-up and neatly permed hair. During the day she had a selection of tailored slacks and expensive cardigans, which the others envied to the extent of making fun of her for being a fussy old maid. But I loved her. She was kind and funny. The only drawback to her bedside visits was the overpowering smell of tobacco from her breath, which a ton of Mint Imperials could not disguise.

Everyone liked Jenny, and when a visitor did actually turn up for her one Saturday we felt like cheering. We three had been in for two months by then. I had visitors every single visiting time – Mum, Dad, brothers, sisters, and even pals at first. Teresa had her weedy wee man on a Saturday and 'as broad as she was long' mother on a Sunday. Until that day, Jenny had had nobody.

There were two of them, both women, really posh-looking and loaded down with tempting-looking parcels. Poor Jenny burst into tears when she saw them.

CHAPTER 2

VISITING TIME AND LETTERS FROM HOME

One of the strange things about being in Law Hospital was, despite the fact that emotions were always just ready to break the surface like a swimmer gulping for air, once one of our friends left – no matter how close they had been – they were hardly missed. It was as if the going back into the outside world had removed any significance that they had had for us. They ceased to exist, apart from being mentioned very occasionally in reminiscences – like long-dead relatives might be.

Was this 'wiping out' a safeguard against coping with too much loss?

Whatever it was, there were always new friends to make and new dramas to observe.

Some of the 'new' friends were my own family. I began to realise that I was getting to know them better now that I was away from them than I had ever done while living under the same roof.

Dad and I had hardly ever had a conversation; now we were in each other's company for at least two hours every week – sometimes three. Since his return from a German POW camp we had never accepted him into the family. The years in between had been important to us as children growing up, and we had accepted not having the presence of a father in our lives – as had most of that generation. He had tried everything to get to know us, to be part of our lives, but to differing degrees we had all rejected him. The eldest of the family, Margaret, had been ten years old when he left; she was fifteen and had started work when he returned. She was too conscious of being 'grown-up' to accept his shows of affection towards her, although she did remember him from before the war. Anna, the second eldest, had been eight and was now thirteen. She did show her enjoyment of his teasing and occasional cuddles, but there are more important things in the life of a thirteen-year-old who has just discovered that boys like her.

Eddie, the eldest son, had been six. He was now eleven, shy and not liking this man taking over his place as his mother's 'man of the house' – except when Dad went to the park and played football with him and his pals. That was OK. Then came Robert, who had been four and did not remember Dad at all. At nine he had the confidence of a twenty-year-old and was acknowledged as the brainbox of the family. He absorbed everything he could learn from this stranger: how to solve crosswords, play Battleships and card games, and how you would always be one step ahead of the next bloke if you got an education.

I was next in the family line. I had been two when we were evacuated to the country at the start of the war. My first memory of Dad was when he returned to the country village where we were 'billeted'. I was seven and expected my daddy to be a kilted red-haired hero, instead of the thin khaki-clad figure who had walked in the door, trying to hug all of us at once. Only Anna and I hugged him back. The others nearly died of embarrassment. From then on I often tried to get his attention away from the others and on to me, but I guess I was just too young to be of interest to him. He did sometimes ask me how I was doing at school, after we moved back to Glasgow, but that was the extent of our communication until I took ill.

When he was told that I had TB he blamed everyone: the doctors, the school and Mum. It was only later that I learned that two of his sisters had died young of the disease.

The first time he visited me on his own I was in a panic, wondering what I could talk about – he had always come with other members of the family before that – yet the time flew past as we discussed books and did a crossword in the magazine he had brought; and he had talked to me about how I would 'take up my education' as soon as I was better. I was the happiest I had ever been since entering that place.

That day set a kind of pattern for visiting hours which lasted until I was discharged – nearly four years later. When Dad came on his own we discussed certain topics. When Mum was with him, or on her own, the conversation would be about family and neighbours and my friends in the ward. With Eddie and Robert, it would be films, music and dancing, and questions about the prettier girls in the ward.

My sisters seldom visited me. Margaret, who had a young baby, did come once or twice, but as the baby was not allowed into the ward I had to speak to them through the window. They were not even allowed into the rec, so it was a bit of a waste of time, although it left me feeling very emotional, knowing I was so dangerous that babies were not allowed near me. The same rules applied to my two younger brothers, Ross and Johnnie, whom I saw only twice in the four years that I was a patient. I began to get an idea how the mothers in the ward must feel, not being allowed to see their children at all.

Anna had moved to London with her new husband, but she kept in touch through letters and parcels. It always made me feel so happily important when Sister Taylor handed them to me with "Another parcel for you, Jean! My, you're a very popular girl!" She seemed to get as much pleasure out of handing them over as I did receiving them. I wish that I could have understood and appreciated her as much then as I do now.

The letters were full of absolutely mad nonsense about bedpans and not being able to sit from having so many injections. I kept them for years and they always made me smile.

CHAPTER 3

WARD 28

In many ways Ward 28 and its occupants were the best introduction any young girl could have to what life is about. Better probably than a boarding school or a term in prison, a nunnery or a primitive female tribe. I say *primitive* because the women in there were ruled by a set of basic values, to which they clung through bad times and good and which they taught me are really all that matters in life.

Their ages varied from early teens, like myself and one or two others, through twenty-to-thirty-odd young marrieds and mothers to middle-aged mothers between forty and fifty plus. There were never any older patients and it didn't take me long to figure that one out: TB did not let people live into old age. And, in those years, many of the young did not get any older and lots of children grew up without mothers – the fight proved too hard for them and TB won again.

Most of us had a fighting chance because of the new drugs, but at first only the worst cases were given the 'wonder drug', and I was one of them. The others had to rely on rest and streptomycin, laced with the fighting spirit which caused the sing-songs and joke-telling that went on every night – even after visiting hours, when most people were a bit down. It was during one of these sing-songs that I had what must have been my first sexual experience (all by myself).

It happened during a kind of initiation rite which every new patient was put through, unless they were too sick or, in my case, too young.

It was a Saturday night after lights-out at nine o'clock. There had been the usual chat about what families and friends were doing in the outside world, much laughter and some crying before the sing-song began. A little Irish girl from Coatbridge, just outside Glasgow, started it off with her version of 'The Rose of Tralee', followed by one of the two spinsters in the ward, Margaret Harriday, a seamstress from Kinning Park (she had been a patient for three years already), who sang a thirties 'weepie' which I had heard Mum singing called 'I Walk Alone'. This brought a few tears and cries of "That was lovely, Margaret!" After that someone would just start up a song and the rest would join in. I kept very quiet – just enjoying listening – for I had been told often enough that singing was not one of my talents.

There was quietness for a few moments and I thought everyone was falling asleep.

Then a voice I couldn't place piped up: "It's time we heard the new lassie singing now, eh, girls?"

"Yeah, it's time."

"Come on, Clara."

"Your turn!" came the chorus and I clutched the blankets around my face and closed my eyes.

I remembered Teresa and Jenny having to sing on their first Saturday in the ward and the threat that was held over them if they refused.

"Sing or get your Malcolm talcummed," the unfamiliar voice called out.

"Wait!" someone else said – I think it was Mary Kelly. "Is the wee lassie sleeping? We don't want to upset the wean."

A tiptoeing figure came crouching down the ward and stopped at my bed. A hand reached out and shook me gently. I kept my eyes tight shut, breathing deeply in a way I thought a soundly sleeping person would. I must have been convincing.

"She's sound asleep" came in a stage whisper from the stealthy figure as she scurried back up the ward like some nocturnal animal searching for food.

The new patient was another Irishwoman. When she had been

shown to her bed on arrival, a few days before, some of the 'girls' had called out cheerfully to her and one of the ward maids had brought her a cup of tea and hung up her clothes for her, but the only response had been a glare and a grunt before she got into her bed and stuck her nose in a newspaper. The only reason they knew her name was that they had heard Sister use it when she came to take down her details and give her a copy of the 'rule book'. She was Clara McCaffery and was not making things easy for herself, with the people she was going to have to live beside for at least a few months. No one had gone home in less than six months at that time.

"Not unless in a box," Margaret Harriday muttered and was hushed by the others in case I heard. They were very protective of me in some ways.

"Right, Clara," a voice called, "everybody that comes into this ward has to sing or we talcum their Malcolm. It's a rule! So what are ye gonnae dae – sing, sing or show yer thing!"

I recognised the voice. It was Kitty – a dying-looking girl of about thirty (although I thought of her as ancient). She had a lovely face, which only seemed to stop smiling when she was coughing agonisingly into her sputum can. Her man came to see her every visiting time and she had shown me photos of her two wee sons, who were as lovely as her. I was shocked that she seemed to be the gang leader.

"Shut up and let people get to sleep! I will not be singing, tonight or any night!"

My teeth were chattering with excitement as I heard the hoarse defiant voice. What would they do to her? What did they mean – talcum your Malcolm? I was sure it must be something really shameful and that 'sing, sing or show your thing' convinced me. Nothing would make me go to sleep now. I had to know what would happen. What if they ever asked me to sing? I was even worse than Jenny and Teresa and they had been awful, but they had sung to avoid having their Malcolm talcummed. It must be something really scary to have frightened a tough wee scruff like Teresa.

A few minutes later I found out, and I still dream about it!

They came running down the ward towards Clara's bed like pyjama-clad birds of prey, brandishing talcum tins and jars like swords above their dishevelled, mad, gorgon-like heads. I could see everything from my blanket peephole. Her bed was only four away from mine. They had checked whether I was sleeping or not before they began their devilish fun. I would have to have been dead to sleep through what happened next. Hands grabbed at the blankets, which Clara was holding up to her chin, and threw them on the floor; others pulled at her pyjama bottoms, but suddenly they stepped back in horror. Why had they stopped?

"Are ye gonnae sing or no?" someone asked in a kind of scared voice.

"I told you. I will not be singing tonight or any night. Do what you like!"

I could see their faces – everyone white and shocked – as she lay back, opened her fat roly-poly legs and challenged them with a look to do their worst. It had totally thrown them. I found out later that they were used to the victim trying desperately to protect her modesty – now they were the embarrassed ones and the ritual was spoiled. Some of them half-heartedly sprinkled some talcum in Clara's direction before wandering back in silence to their own beds.

There was no more singing that night.

My reaction to the experience was to wet my pyjamas. Only much later did I realise it was not with urine. I had had my first sexual arousal – thanks to a fat Irishwoman!

Those first few months in the sanatorium were like some sort of strange holiday from normal life – well, what had been normal for me. I spent a lot of the time sleeping, or pretending to sleep, except at visiting times or when Jenny or Teresa came to my bed to talk to me. Teresa was hating almost everything about the place now that she was feeling better. She told us that she had never had so much to eat in her life.

"Mind you, I would like it if we got mair chips," she said, "and could have a fag without hidin' in the cludgie. But at least I can go for a wee walk wi' ma Jimmy when he comes up. He says he's gonnae take me to the woods on Saturday." She gave a dirty laugh and was glared at by Jenny. I had no idea why. She also complained about the number of baths she was being given: "I think some of they nurses are queer," she said, "and just like touching my body." Another dirty laugh was followed by a glare from Jenny, who walked away in disgust.

At last I began to get over the embarrassment of being in bed in front of all those strangers and took some notice of the patients on either side and those across the ward from me.

Next to Teresa – directly facing me – was Betty Hughes; next to her was Cathy Brannigan. I couldn't make out the person after that, for a pillar obscured my view. Beside me, on my left, was Margaret Harriday, and two beds away Mrs Alexander. These five people, plus Jenny and the nurses, made up my social circle at the start of my stay at Law Hospital. They had one thing in common – they were all living under the threat of an early death from TB. Apart from that, one could not have met six more different characters, or stranger company for a thirteen-year-old girl.

Betty Hughes was the eldest in one of those families that were said to 'have it in the family'. Her mother had died of TB while being nursed at home by Betty, her three sisters and her brother. She had refused to go into hospital – not realising that her presence at home was sentencing her family to the same fate as herself.

When Betty had been diagnosed, people shook their heads and said, "It must be in the family – her mother died of it, after all."

At that time it was seen as a curse passed down through the generations, not as a highly contagious disease which was preventable if the right precautions were taken.

The Hughes family were amazing: every visiting day one or other of the three sisters would appear, sometimes accompanied by the old father, whose wheeze could be heard throughout the ward like music in some eerie chimney, but always accompanied by the brother, Jimmy – an ugly-looking red-haired lad with the ghastly white face that some redheads have, yet his expression of good humour and concern for his sister cancelled out his odd appearance. He spoke in a high girlish voice and his sisters called him 'oor big Jessie', but it was obvious that they loved him and were proud of him. He worked in a gent's outfitter's.

Betty told us with a giggle, "He loves his work, the big Jessie!"

I learned so much about love just by watching that family, and I have never forgotten them and their tragic story, which had only just begun, with the mother's death.

Jimmy arrived on his own one Saturday and Sister Taylor followed him in. Then she and Ellen, the orderly, put screens around Betty's bed. I have to admit, I was thrilled by the excitement and drama of it all. The ward seemed to suddenly become silent, and even the visitors at other beds could not keep from looking towards the screens. Only when patients were really ill were their beds screened, and the belief was that Betty was coming on really well on the 'wonder drug'. What was happening behind that beige curtain?

How can I describe the sound that escaped from that screen and made people grab each other's hands as if for safety from the horror of it? It was like a baby's cry – a tortured baby – a baby whose heart was breaking.

Then came Betty's voice: "Oh, naw, Jimmy, not oor Mary. Naw, naw, please, not oor Mary!"

And Sister's voice: "Now now, dear, you must be strong. She's young. She'll be all right. Please keep calm."

When Jimmy left and the screens were taken away, Betty was lying on her back with the covers pulled up to her face; only her eyes, with swollen red lids, were showing. At first nobody dared to approach her, then Kitty walked down the ward, looking neither right nor left, and made straight for Betty's bed. With a funny little jump she sat up on the bed – a cardinal sin in Sister's eyes – and, laying her head down on the pillow, put her arms around the other girl and began to talk quietly to her. None of us heard what she said, and when Sister came into the ward she looked sadly at them, but let them be.

We learned that yet another of the Hughes family had fallen victim to the 'curse' – the sister next to Betty in age, but quite a bit younger. She was a big-busted, rosy-faced, strong-looking girl of about eighteen – a picture of health, but her chest X-ray, which all of the family got at regular intervals, showed a shadow on her lung and she was to join her sister in hospital.

"They say it's just a precaution, just to be on the safe side," Betty said to anyone and everyone, although it seemed she was really talking to herself.

Big Mary was an asset to the ward – making everybody laugh with her stories about 'fellas at the dancing' and the number of rollers she wore in her hair every night, making people ask the question 'How on earth does she sleep with that lot in her head?' She was nothing like Betty, who was a serious person, given to reading her prayer book and telling her rosary beads, which I loved to watch as I had never seen such a thing before – I wished I was a Roman Catholic, for a time.

Jimmy now divided the hour of visiting time between his two sisters. If he was on his own, he spent a half-hour with each of them; if one or other of the sisters was with him, they swapped seats at half-time, until one of the nurses asked Sister if it was all right for Mary to sit by Betty's bed during visiting hour – a request which was reluctantly granted.

Betty's 'bed mate' on the other side from Teresa – Cathy Brannigan – was the weirdest person I had ever come across. I thought of her as middle-aged, which meant she was about twenty-four and had nothing attractive about her appearance. Her hair was colourless, lank and greasy, framing a big face, with a long greyhound-like nose and a mouth like a subway tunnel full of huge off-white teeth – poor girl! But with the cruelty of my thirteen years I found her repulsive and ignored her attempts at friendship by often pretending to be tired or even asleep when she visited my bedside, usually carrying a box of sweets, a comic or some fruit. I couldn't help myself – I just didn't like looking at her.

Her visitors were very posh when she had any, which was not all that often. I don't think she had a mother, because it was only her father and an aunt who ever came. I had the habit (I still have it) of comparing people to characters from fiction. Cathy's father was Mr Jarndyce from *Bleak House* and the aunt was Betsy

Trotwood in modern dress – Dickens was my favourite author then.

Cathy was another one of the guinea pigs for the 'wonder drug', and for a while it seemed to be working for her. Sister told her one morning, as she brought round the mail, that she was to be allowed to go outside for a short walk in the afternoons, weather permitting.

"Why don't you go out with your father when he comes on Saturday?" she smiled.

But Cathy only gave one of her horrible snuffly laughs and said, "He won't be up for a few weeks. He's away on business. I'll manage by myself."

It's only now I realise how sad that claim was, because we never saw any of her visitors for months after that, and by the time they did appear she had been moved to a 'cubicle' – one-bed rooms at either side of the corridor leading into the ward – where patients were taken to die so as not to distress the other patients.

Still, she did have a short time to enjoy her walks, her outdoor clothes (a long tweed coat with about 100 buttons down the front and a woolly hat she had knitted herself, which looked as if one of the seven dwarves should be wearing it) causing much sniggering behind her back, particularly from me.

She came back from one of her walks about ten minutes after she had left and got into her bed without coming to visit me, for which I was shamefully glad. The visitors had all left the ward and we were just sitting, waiting for our afternoon tea, looking at what had been brought to us – books, chocolates and Lucozade for me – when Cathy suddenly sat straight up in bed and grabbed for her sputum can from the locker. I wanted to look away! She was coughing and laughing at the same time and looking into the can (as she always did). Betty and Teresa saw the look of horror on my face and turned to look at what was causing it. I had never seen blood so red. At first I thought she was having a bad nosebleed. Then she lifted her face and looked directly at me. She seemed to be grinning like some ecstatic vampire. I had seen the old black-and-white movie of *Dracula*, and here it was in front of me in ‘glorious Technicolor’. The blood spouted through her teeth in thick gobbets and suddenly, with one horrible rattling cough, overflowed – like a dam bursting – on to the white bed mat.

Betty was the first to move. She got out of bed and ran out of the ward, calling for a nurse to “Come quickly – Cathy’s pourin’ wi’ blood. Oh, somebody come!”

Within seconds, Sister Taylor and two of the nurses were there, dragging the screens around Cathy’s bed and helping Betty back into hers.

In the morning there was a freshly made-up empty bed where Cathy’s had been, and I felt sure that she had died in the night. There had been a lot of coming and going behind the screens, even after lights-out, but I had kept my head under the blankets and eventually fell asleep to the sound of Cathy’s laugh/cough, whispering voices and the soft squeak of rubber-soled shoes.

She didn’t die that time. She had been put into the side room in preparation for the main event, which was two months in coming.

My ‘neighbour’ Margaret Harriday was another of the long-serving patients, for whom the ‘wonder drug’ was the last hope. She had been in other sanatoriums before Law Hospital and altogether – she told me – she had been in for four years – in Law Hospital for two of those. She had been moved from the last one, in Perthshire, to be closer for her mother (who was her only relative) to visit. She was lucky in a way – most of those who had been there for a number of years seldom got visitors. If they had families and friends they seemed to have forgotten them. I felt quite smug because I had someone at my bedside every visiting day (a wee quiet voice sometimes asked me what had happened to my pals after the first few weeks, but I supposed their mothers wouldn’t let them visit – after all, Law Hospital was ‘away in the wilds’.

Margaret was in her late thirties, she said when the subject of age came up, but she acted like someone from another era. She wore her long grey hair up in ‘sweeps’ at the side and put on pancake make-up and red lipstick every morning, after she was washed, repairing it several times during the day. Her figure was quite buxom, with a slim waist which she showed off by belting her dressing gown very tightly and wearing fitted trousers and sweaters when she had her ‘up’ time. She had her own teeth, of which she was very proud, and gave me hints on how to look after mine.

“Men don’t like girls with false teeth,” she told me with one of her little-girl giggles.

I had never met anybody like her before, with her fussiness about her appearance and keeping her bed and locker tidy. Jenny told me she was ‘a typical old maid’, but she reminded me more of a schoolteacher I had had in primary school and maybe that explained my respect for her and her advice. She was actually very pretty when you got past the old-fashioned hairstyle and make-up. She showed me photos of herself looking like one of those 1930s film stars – in a one-piece bathing costume, with her hair in exactly the same style, although jet black, and I struggled to hide my amazement.

“I bet you had loads of boyfriends.” I said, bringing a smile to her lips and a tear to her eyes.

The ‘wonder drug’ seemed to be working with her, and she confided that she expected to be moved to the convalescent ward “after my next check-up”. I did wonder why she was kept at ‘our’ end of the ward, which was accepted to be for very ill patients, but at least I managed to keep the thought to myself.

One bed beyond Margaret was Mrs Alexander – I never heard anyone calling her by her Christian name – in fact, if I did know it I cannot remember it. She was just one of those women who are always called by their married name.

She was a bed-patient like me and had to suffer the humiliation of bed baths and bedpans, although, unlike the rest of us, the nurses would screen her bed when she had to have a pee or a bowel movement (as I learned to refer to that basic necessity). I suppose she gave me my first experience of snobbery. She visibly shuddered when the ward maids told harmless smutty jokes, as they did regularly. They kept everyone (apart from Mrs Alexander) laughing as they washed and polished everything that didn’t move and some things that did. It was the only light relief most of the patients had, but Mrs Alexander hated it and showed her disapproval by tutting and even complaining to Sister, who had the offender in the duty room for 'a good talking to' without any effect whatever.

What was her reason for being snobbish? Her man was head rep for a confectionery firm, had a company car (most of our families had never owned a car and had little hope of ever doing so in the 1950s), travelled all over the country and wore made-to-measure suits. She had never worked since she married him. They had no children and he tried to satisfy her every whim as if she was mistress to his slave.

He was friendly and always had a cheerful word for us girls in the surrounding beds, even bringing me packets of butterscotch every time he visited. She smirked smugly as if his friendliness was something that she allowed from the goodness of her heart, but I was sure she hated it and felt he was lowering himself by talking to us. That made me twice as happy to get the butterscotch.

As I got stronger I began to enjoy things about my strange life. I had never had so much attention in all of my thirteen years: colourful tops and cardigans to wear over the hospital pyjamas, which were like cartoon convict suits and ten sizes too big, more sweets and fruit than our whole family had had in several Christmases, talcum powder, perfume, books and magazines, letters, cards and parcels through the post, and – best of all – the company of my mother and father three times a week and my brothers on alternate Saturdays. When people say that I lost precious years of my life in hospital I don't agree. I gained more than I lost.

CHAPTER 4

RESULTS DAYS

Apart from the brave jokes, sing-songs and talk about men there were other things that helped us to survive in the unreal (but sometimes too real) world of the sanatorium. When I look back at them I think of them as 'events'.

Every six weeks a different group of patients was taken to the X-ray block – an event in itself – and had to wait a week for the results, which would then be given to them in a private consultation with Dr Ballantine or his wife, Dr Morton. Friday was the day for both X-rays and results, although on results days no group went for an X-ray, so there was a fortnight between the 'ceremonies'.

Fridays, particularly results days, were even more exciting than the weekend visiting days. Because of the closeness of the relationships which existed among us as a group, the anticipation of the doctors' verdicts swept us all along in a rip tide of nerves. X-ray days were more about getting dolled up for any good-looking radiographers who might be on duty, or maybe even a light flirtation with the ambulance driver or (if really desperate) a hospital porter, but results days were about stomach-churning nerves, black disappointment, tears and elation. I've never experienced anything I could compare to those days – never!

Another event happened every Monday evening – Film Night!

Those who were allowed out of bed could attend a film being shown in the rec, which was a ward converted for recreational activities, just across the corridor from Ward 28 – our ward. Once in a blue moon a concert party would come and perform there, but, mostly, Film Night was its only use.

For the first few months I was not allowed the treat of Film Night and then – I'll never forget it – Sister came to my bed on a Monday after tea, all blushes and excitement, like a young girl telling her pal she had a date.

"Dr Morton says you're well enough to have a little treat, Jean. Get yourself tidied up. . . ." She paused and looked around at the adjoining beds as if to make sure she had an audience for her announcement. "You're going to the films. Put on your best bib and tucker!"

Just as she finished speaking, Nurse McKinnon wheeled an ancient wooden wheelchair up to my bed and began putting some of my pillows on to it. Sister opened my 'wardrobe' and took out one of my new cardigans – a white angora with embroidery on the front.

"This looks warm and pretty," she actually giggled, "like Cinderella going to the ball! I'll leave you to it, Nurse. Enjoy yourself, Jean."

I hadn't time to be nervous about my first night out for about six months. Nurse McKinnon had me dressed and in the ancient transport before I had time to consider that the stern Sister Taylor was obviously a young girl at heart and was taking as much pleasure from the surprise 'event' as I was.

After that I was taken to the films every week – in my chariot – until my matchstick legs were strong enough to carry me. It was there that I was first kissed and cuddled by a girl – I liked it.

Farewells were other eventful occasions that happened fairly frequently, for as the treatment of the disease was begun earlier, and the drugs became more effective, long-term stays became the exception rather than the norm, so the farewell events became almost regular in their frequency. The main reason for patients being discharged was that the disease had been, as Dr Morton put it, stopped in its tracks and, with good care, would never return. It was always emphasised that the drugs and treatments did not 'cure' TB, but stopped it spreading and repaired most of the damage it had caused.

"Remember," she would tell patients who were ready to go home, "you have been damaged and must always take care of yourself if you want to remain fit and healthy: no late nights, no smoking and plenty of good food and rest."

The other reason for patients being sent home still led to the farewell ceremony, but it was a veil made of shouts of "Good luck!" and affectionate hugs, which covered the secret that we all knew but did not let on about: these were the women and girls who were being sent home to die. They were beyond treatment. The drugs had come too late for them. No matter how few late nights or how good the food and rest, the disease would win the battle.

There were other farewells, but they were unspoken, to those who died in the ward – usually in a cubicle like the one into which Cathy Brannigan had been taken after that bloody drama, which I can still see after all these years. It is, in a way, more vivid to me now than it was to that thirteen-year-old girl. I did see Cathy just before the mortuary trolley came for her in the middle of the night. That sight will never leave my memory.

My pal from the ambulance – Teresa – was not officially passed fit and ready for home, but she decided to say farewell anyway. She told Margaret Harriday and me, after one visiting day, that her man was "fed up sleepin' on his own. He says he'll look for somebody else if I'm in here much longer. He says I don't look as if there's anythin' wrong wi' me and I can get the same drugs frae ma ain doctor as I'm gettin' in here."

Margaret told her she was a fool and would be back, worse than ever, in a few weeks, but she just said, "I don't want tae lose ma man. I'm goin' to sign myself out."

And she did, the very next day. She saw Dr Morton in the morning, and the wee weed she was married to came and collected her that afternoon. He stood at the entrance to the ward, sneering as she made her rounds to say goodbye, and dragged her out carrying her own suitcase.

Betty Hughes was the next one to leave. The 'wee daddy' was

ill and she felt that her sisters were too young to look after him – besides, they were still at school and Jimmy had to work to support them all. The doctors let her go reluctantly, warning her that she must attend the clinic, put in for a home help and take things as easy as possible. I think they knew that all their good work with her would be undone, but also that she would sign herself out if they did not agree. Her sister, Big Mary, stayed behind and we were all crying watching them saying goodbye, as Jimmy, with his red hair standing on end, his face marred with red blotches against his usual pastiness, stood waiting to take her home.

The farewell ceremony was not always such a sad affair. For those leaving because they were 'cured' it was a mixture of sadness, happiness and mostly relief to get back into their lives. There was a certain pattern to it, which someone had started in the past and which was now stuck to quite rigidly.

It actually began just after the evening bedtime drink, about eight o'clock. The lucky woman, or sometimes women, would pass round sweets, cakes or biscuits which one of the orderlies had been commissioned to bring in, and we would all tuck in – laughing and talking in quavery voices, with tears in them. I thought of the midnight feasts described in some of my schoolgirl books and, being delighted at the excitement of it all, had to fake the sadness that the others seemed to feel. It was not until I was much older that I understood how you can be happy and sad at the same time.

The next part of the farewell took place after lights-out, when there was a special sing-song. The person leaving always sang (some of them were awful) and there were no threats of Malcolm-talcumming, although there was a lot of leaping in and out of each other's beds and dirty laughter, until the night nurse came in, shining her torch around and telling us it was time to go to sleep in a voice which she failed to make stern and authoritative.

"Come on, you lot. It'll soon be morning. You married women that are leaving in the morning'll not get much sleep tomorra night" was followed by a dirty laugh, which echoed around the ward.

Home patients usually left around eleven o'clock, after morning tea and the Doctor's rounds, and that's when the real tears were shed – even by me.

The patients who were leaving visited each bed in turn, being given cards, gifts and 'all the bests', depending on the strength of the friendship they had had with the occupant of the bed. There were tears, laughter and suggestive remarks – most of which went over my head, although I laughed as knowingly as the rest – but there was a look of fear on many of the happy faces. Looking back, I realise it was a twofold fear: fear that maybe they would never be the one saying farewell and going back into the world and fear for those who were leaving. Please, God, their expressions said, please, don't let them come back! Those who did come back – and there were still quite a few – came back for a less happy farewell.

Betty Hughes was one of those, as was poor Teresa. Betty was wheeled back after three months of 'freedom' – straight into a cubicle to cry her way into a painful death. Teresa was admitted to another ward: the TB had spread to her spine. She died alone; her man had got tired of visiting her and nobody else in her family ever appeared.

The first time that I was taken out of the ward for an X-ray (before that they brought in a portable contraption and X-rayed me in bed; I can still feel the metallic chill of the plate that was placed between me and my pillows as the radiographer said, "Breath in, hold it, breath out" – words I heard many times in the next four years) I was sitting up, dressed in my best cardigan and the new black trousers my mother had brought for the time when I would become an up-patient. As soon as I was bathed Nurse McKinnon had taken me to the bathroom, before the breakfast dishes were even cleared away. She had washed my hair and given me a 'finger-wave', which – she assured me – made me look like a 'wee china doll'. I put on pale-pink lipstick and a generous dusting of face powder. I had an hour to wait, but I was ready, as were the other four patients in the group. We looked as if we were going on a big date or for a screen test (I'd read about them in my film books), and the others perched on my bed with me until Sister came in and shooed them off like a farmer's wife chasing her hens.

The ambulance ride to the X-ray block was very different from the last one I had been on, when I entered Law Hospital for the first time. Everyone was talking at once and laughing at nothing, and the reek of talcum powder and perfume made me sneeze. There was one similarity – Jenny Christie was once again a fellow passenger. The others were Margaret Harriday, Mary Hughes and a new patient, Ina Wright, a girl of about sixteen.

Ina became my pal after that day, and we kept in touch even after we were home, until she moved away and I couldn't find her.

Margaret and Jenny were trying to maintain the dignity that befitted 'grown-ups', but they could not resist laughing at Mary's outrageous jokes and suggestive banter with the driver and the young nurse who made up the party. I had a sudden memory of the 'bus runs' that people in our street back in Govan used to organise – usually to Ayr or Saltcoats – and I felt the same excitement with which the anticipation of going to the seaside had filled me at going to the X-ray unit, enclosed in a box on wheels, with these perfumed and painted women.

We had to walk a few yards down a brown-painted corridor to get to the X-ray unit – past two male wards. A porter with greasy hair and a blue chin pushed me in a wheelchair, taking great care to make sure that my feet were placed safely on the step. This meant he had to handle my knees and thighs quite a bit, which caused Mary and Ina to nearly burst with excitement and Jenny and Margaret to hold their heads up as if they were not aware of the shouts and whistles from the men in the wards. Ina told me afterwards that her pants 'were soaking', but I thought she was just desperate to get to the toilet for a pee. Was I really as naive as that?

The excitement lasted until teatime and even, in Mary's case, bedtime as she told the other patients how she and Ina had 'waved to the men and blew them kisses'.

"I bet we caused a few wet dreams to the frustrated souls," she said, laughing like the laughing clown in the fairground. Her meaning was lost on me!

We had a full week to wait for results day, which was another occasion for those taking part to get dolled up. Ina had on very tight black trousers and a pink-and-white striped T-shirt, which showed off her amazing bust (I was green with envy every time I compared them to my 'knots in thread') and her dry-looking reddish hair, the colour of a coconut shell, was frizzed to resemble a rusty-pot cleaner. She was not a pretty girl, yet any males who came into the ward – porters, radiographers and such – looked at her as if she were a meal on a plate and they hadn't eaten for days. Oh, how I envied her – everyone treated me like a wee girl!

Margaret Harriday had her hair up in sweeps, like an old-time film star, perfectly made up and wearing one of the 'feather and shell' patterned jumpers her old mother knitted for her. I felt sorry for the hope in her eyes, which she was trying to hide by assuming a casual, uncaring manner – which fooled no one.

Big Mary had on the whole shebang: nylons, high-heeled shoes, a tight, straight skirt and a gorgeous green satin blouse with 'bishop's sleeves'. It was as if she was dressed ready to be given the all-clear for home already, but the impression was spoiled by her shaky voice and feverish complexion – she was scared to death of what was waiting for her in that consulting room. We all were.

Jenny Christie, with her neat hair, discreet lipstick and buttoned-up shirt-blouse, looked like the prim, efficient office worker that she was.

I was being allowed to walk – with a nurse on one arm and an orderly on the other – the short distance from my bed to the duty room where Dr Morton or her husband, Dr Ballantine, awaited us with our results. For the occasion I was wearing the pale-blue twinset Mum had brought in for me and my new black trousers, and Nurse McKinnon had waved my hair in the 'china doll' style. I couldn't eat my breakfast, although it was my favourite – two fingers of toast with a bit of bacon and a slice of tomato on each – so I was glad to hold their arms to stop me keeling over from weakness and excitement.

Jenny's name was called first and we all shouted, "Good luck!" as she left the main part of the ward.

For the first time I noticed how curved her spine was – making her look like a tortoise with its head poking out of its shell – and the way she lurched when she walked, as if she would break into a run at any moment. I hated myself for noticing these things about my friend, but I was not in control of what my eyes told me. She was not with the Doctor for long and, as the ritual dictated, she stopped on entering the ward and gave the verdict.

"Much the same as last time," she said, giving a funny little laugh. "Progress is slow, but there is an improvement and she wants to see me putting on another stone at least before considering discharging me." She shook her head and walked slowly towards her bed. "I've never put on weight in my life. I guess I'll have to cheat the next time they weigh me."

She shrugged and laughed when she said this, as if to show us that it didn't bother her, but I'm sure I was not the only one who saw through her brave act. What could anybody say?

Big Mary was next. She came swaggering down the ward as if it was Saturday night and she was going to the Barrowland Ballroom looking for a lumber.

"This is it, girls," she said as she left the ward. "This time next week I'll be strollin' down Sauchiehall Street wi' ma pals."

She looked half her usual size when she came out, but she soon had everybody laughing, saying, "I'm completely cured, but they're keeping me for a wee while longer to cheer you lot up and Sister Taylor disnae want me to go."

A few people laughed. No one asked her what she had really heard in the duty room. That night, after lights-out, the women nearest her heard her crying and one of them went to comfort her and the whole story came out: Betty had had a really bad setback and was coming back to Law Hospital. The father was still unwell and Dr Morton had told Mary that, although she was almost ready to be discharged, they would not let her go until arrangements were made for someone to look after him. (Some of the women said – not to Mary – that he should be in a home.) They refused to discharge another sister for her to be brought back 'worse than ever', as Betty was, as we soon saw.

Margaret Harriday kept up her ladylike bearing, not hurrying, holding her head high. She had a smile on her lips like a mother wears when she's indulging her child's silly behaviour, yet I couldn't shake off a sadness that came over me as I gave her a little wave when she passed my bed.

"Everything's going fine," she said. "The drugs are doing their job. They said it won't be much longer now. They just have to be sure that my strength is built up enough before they let me go. I've to take another half-hour of exercise time. It's a good result. I'm delighted with it."

I had never heard anyone expressing delight in such a sad voice or with tears in their eyes, yet we all took her word for it – as far as we showed her anyway. She had been a patient for just over three years and I wondered how much longer she could bear it. When her old mother visited that weekend, they were whispering and holding hands most of the time. Margaret seemed to be comforting the old lady and – young and daft as I was – I wondered who would comfort Margaret.

Ina came out beaming and giggling. Her news was good.

"She says the drugs are beginning to work already. I've only been on them a month and they're amazed at my progress." She was putting on a posh voice when she repeated the Doctor's words, but reverted to her Glaswegian twang as she continued: "Ah've no tae overdo it, but ah have to go out for walks in the grounds and help with any wee light jobs in the ward. She says ah'll be moved tae the convalescent ward after ma course is finished and providing there's a bed." Turning her attention to me: "Come on, hen, you're next. She said to send you in. Ah bet you get good news tae."

Staff Nurse Brown (more of her later) came and offered me the support of one of her arms; Ina took the other side and escorted me to the duty room. I felt as if I was making an entrance onstage and the fluttering in my stomach reinforced the feeling.

Dr Morton smiled and told me to sit down opposite her across the desk. She sat looking at me for a full minute before coming around to stand in front of me.

"Well, my dear," she said, "how are you feeling?" Not waiting for an answer: "A lot better than when you first came in, I bet, eh?"

Something about her manner was jangling my nerves. Something was wrong! She felt the sides of my neck and peered into my eyes.

"Don't look so worried," she said with a gentle laugh meant to reassure, but only making me feel worse. "Your X-ray shows a big improvement. You're responding well to the treatment and Sister tells me you've put on a little bit of weight, but still not enough. You must eat up all of your meals to build up your strength."

Oh, my God, what was all this leading up to?

"There's another form of treatment that Dr Ballantine and I think will be really good for you, but I'm afraid it means continuing to be a bed-patient for a little bit longer."

Did she know the effect her words were having on me? She was still smiling as she went back to sit at the desk. I had been so sure that I was finished for good with bedpans and all the other embarrassments of being a bed-patient, that she could not have made me feel worse if she had said my X-ray showed the disease had spread. Maybe it had and this 'new treatment' was just to cover up the fact. What about being allowed to go to the toilet myself, have baths, wash my hair and go to Film Night? it was too much to see all of these being placed out of reach.

I burst into tears and cried out, "How can you say I'm getting better and then say you're keeping me a bed-patient?"

Sister Taylor must have heard me from outside the door. Suddenly she was there by my side, hushing me as if she was afraid I might upset the Doctor. Between them they quietened me and then she described the treatment, which started me crying in earnest.

"I'm going to explain a little bit about what's been happening to you, Jean," she began. (I could see through the ploy of talking to me as if I were an adult, and took it as a compliment.) "When you were first diagnosed, both your lungs were very badly affected. You were a very sick young lady, as I'm sure you know. But since being on the course of drugs that Dr Ballantine and I prescribed, plus bed rest and good food, you have come on like a house on fire, and quite a lot of that is down to the great wee fighter you've shown yourself to be. What we're asking is that you keep up that spirit and help us to finally make you healthier than you've ever been." She paused to consult my case notes, which were open on her desk, and exchange a 'funny' look with Sister Taylor. "Now, Jean, what has been happening is this: your right lung is healing up really well, with just the treatment so far, but your left lung needs a bit more help, and that's what this new treatment is about. It involves raising the foot of your bed on blocks and you lying on your left side as much as possible so that your right lung does all the work and your left gets complete rest. After six weeks we take you down and, hopefully, you will be ready for getting up and about – in stages, of course. Another patient will be undergoing the same treatment, so we'll put you together and you can keep each other cheerful. Sister will take you back to your bed now. Keep that fighting spirit, my dear – the porters will put your beds up tomorrow."

What were my feelings about what I saw as a setback? I was nearly fourteen – still a wean in many ways. I was disappointed, yet kind of thrilled that I was being 'selected' for this new treatment and feeling kind of superior at being talked to as an adult – that had never happened to me before! I regretted that I would not be going to Film Night for a while, but her words about my 'great fighting spirit' made me feel kind of heroic – like Grace Darling or Joan of Arc. The physical difficulties did not really strike me at first, so I re-entered the ward with a kind of glow of courage in the face of adversity, shining from my tear-filled eyes. Bette Davis could not have done better.

The porters came early the next morning, joking as they raised the ends of our beds that "You'll no be able tae get up tae any mischief for a while, eh?" although they were obviously sorry for us. I had made sure that I'd had a real bath and used the lavatory before being imprisoned (that was how I had started to think of it). Six weeks is a long time when you're young – it's only as you get older that time flies.

At first it was good being the centre of sympathetic attention from everyone – the other patients, the nurses, ward maids and, above all, my visitors. Dad began to come twice a week – Saturdays and Wednesdays; Mum came on Sundays and sometimes Saturdays with Dad; my two elder brothers came every second Sunday; and my sisters came whenever they could. My younger brothers were not allowed to visit and my school pals had either lost interest or were forbidden by their parents – after all, I did have a contagious disease. Anyway, the presents Dad brought me – mostly books – and the good things to eat that Mum brought made up for the others not coming. I did not miss them – even my two closest pals. They were irrelevant to this new world into which I had been thrust. Ina Wright was my best pal now, and in the years to come many more friends popped in and out of my life.

The other patient undergoing the torture – as I thought of it – was a dark, angry-looking woman who seemed old to me: an ancient twenty-nine. Her name was Rachel and she was married to an equally dark and angry-looking man, called Donald. I have two vivid memories of her: she did not stick to the treatment – lying on your side at all times except when using a bedpan, eating or being washed – and whenever Donald visited I was aware that his hands were beneath the blankets and she was wriggling about and whimpering. I saw this accidentally the first time and tried to avoid looking in their direction after that, which was difficult as they were directly in my line of vision as I lay on my left side. If I had no visitors, I would close my eyes and pretend to sleep or use a book as a screen between us. When I did have visitors, I talked incessantly to hold their attention. The thought of any of my family seeing their antics made me break out in a sweat. Yet sometimes the voyeur in me won and I would sneak a look at them from behind my book. I got the same feeling of pleasurable horror as I had experienced when I saw my first 'dirty drawing', which some boys had passed round our classroom.

I had other feelings to occupy me. For the first time in my life I experienced depression, although I was too young to have a name for it. I wonder if this is how animals in cages feel – watching life going on, but not being part of it; seeing the looks of curiosity and pity as free beings walk by or stand and stare. I was not behind bars, but I was not part of the life beyond the end of my bed. This was going to be the longest six weeks of my life. I tried to cheer myself up by remembering that school holidays lasted eight weeks and they were over just when you were beginning to enjoy your freedom, but nothing worked.

In Glasgow there is a saying to describe someone or something that really gets you down: 'Would that no sicken your happiness?' Well, my happiness was truly sickened and I felt that it would never recover.

As well as the foreplay going on in the next bed, my bowels and my stomach refused to adjust to being permanently on a slope, so that I was either being fed what is the most disgusting concoction known to man – liquid paraffin and cascara – by Sister Taylor (wearing a look that said, "This hurts me more than it hurts you") or being given enemas. Whatever dignity I had developed in my fourteen years was destroyed by the bodily intrusion and embarrassment of having soapy water injected into my rectum via a red rubber tube and then waiting in terror for the bubbling and gurgling from my insides that told me I was about to 'go' and yelling for a bedpan.

After two weeks was up, I had given up begging the nurses to have my bed put back down, and gave in to the black cloud that pervaded me. Other patients – even those whom I thought of as friends – gave up stopping by my bed to cheer me up, apart from Ina, who chatted away to me, telling me of her upbringing, without demanding any response. My visitors sometimes had to sit through the hour without a word from me. It was like being in a huff with the world and I could not come out of it. The fighting spirit that Dr Morton had so admired had shrivelled up and died at the first real challenge.

Another two weeks went by under the black cloud. Then, suddenly, the disgusting Rachel said something which made it begin to clear: "Just another two weeks," I heard her say to Donald as she was saying goodbye at the end of visiting time, "and then I'll be up and able to go over to the rec with you – or even outside."

I didn't hear his reply as it was muffled by the slurping suction of her lips.

Two weeks! I was two-thirds of the way through my sentence. My spirit was off the canvas and on its feet with its dukes up. I could stand another two weeks all right!

The portable X-ray machine was trundled into the ward a week before we were due to 'get down', and we knew that by the following Friday – results day – we would know whether the six weeks of misery had been worth it. I was confident it would be in my case, because I had really stuck to the rules of lying constantly on my left side – not that I was especially conscientious, but the depression was making me totally lethargic and uninterested in sitting up to look at the 'outside world'.

I was not so sure about Rachel, who had often broken the rules – even sneaking up to use the toilet once during the night, when the night nurse was occupied with another patient, at the top end of the ward.

So much for being smug: Rachel emerged from her consultation with the Doctor waving her arms in ecstasy, whereas I stumbled out in tears.

The six weeks had made no difference to my left lung. I would no longer be on 'complete bed rest', but I had to undergo still more treatment before I would be an up-patient. This disappointment made me feel lower than knowing that girls – like Betty Hughes and Cathy Brannigan – had died young and in pain.

I was fourteen years old.

CHAPTER 5

INA

There were so many sad stories, and hearing them developed my attitude to life for ever after. In some ways they made me old beyond my years, but, mainly, they gave me an insight into how many women were deprived of their right to a decent life and how others seemed to suffer so many blows that should have crushed the spirit out of them, yet they could still put in their curlers at night and paint their lips in the morning – ready to meet the next blow with a brave face. No boxer ever rose from the canvas to fight again as many times as those women. At the age of fourteen they showed me the greatness of the human spirit.

One of the first stories I was allowed to know was Ina Wright's.

We became really close pals when my bed was put up on 'stilts'. I was so down and, looking back, I realise how good she was to persevere in her efforts to cheer me up and just think about the fun we would have when the six weeks were over and, even further ahead, when "We'll be outta this place and goin' tae the dancin' and out wi' fellas an' that," as she put it, giving me a big hug that crushed me against her lovely soft breasts.

It was during one of these 'cheering-up' sessions that she began to tell me about her upbringing in the Partick district of Glasgow. As she revealed the experiences of her seventeen years (More than most people suffer in seventy years) I had my eyes and my mind opened so thoroughly that, I'm sure, my dad would have removed me from the hospital if he had known about it.

Ina had been born to a mother who was – she said this without a blush – ‘a bit of a good thing’. No one knew who the father was and nobody cared. Ina was quickly offloaded on to her granny, ‘the auld bitch’, who brought her up to know how a slap can make your ears ring and a ‘good belting’ can put you off sitting down for a week at a time.

What amazed me more than hearing about the beatings (the most I had ever had was a wee slap on the legs) was the way Ina laughed as she told me about them. She seemed to think there was nothing wrong about them. It was as if she assumed that it was like that for everybody. When I told her that my brothers and sisters and I were never ‘given the belt’, she said, “You must be a lot of goody-goodies, then.”

She asked me if I’d ever ‘had it’, and I turned scarlet and said, “I’m too young and, anyway, my mum says you should never let a boy near you ’til you’re married.”

What a prissy little prude I must have seemed to her, with her loads of sexual experience, which she enjoyed describing to me.

“You should see the look on your wee face!” she would laugh, and pinch my burning cheek, as she gave me her sex-education lessons.

She had started off by giving the boys at her primary school ‘a feel’ on top of her knickers, and then a quick look up the leg, and finally a ‘real feel’ and even, for those she liked, ‘a real good look’. She was the most popular lassie in the school at first and then they had all started taking a rise out of her.

“They came into the lassies’ shed one day and just grabbed me,” she said, looking unusually sad. “It was the bigger lads and they were too strong for me. They pulled aff ma knickers and put them in the bin an’ then they paraded me round the playground wi’ ma skirt right up – you could see everything and the lassies were a’ laughin’ as well – even ma pals – until a teacher came out and chased them aff me. But it was me that got the belt and sent hame wi’ a note for ma granny.”

I’m sure the sickness I felt showed in my face.

“You a’ right, hen?” she asked with a return of her mad grin. “Don’t worry – I got ma revenge on every one o’ them before long.”

She didn't tell me then how she got her revenge. That story was saved for another day, but I was free to imagine – and could I imagine! My imagination helped me to get through the years that followed.

The strange thing about Ina was that she wanted to love everybody and for them to love her back. I got first-hand experience of this trait the first time I was allowed to attend Film Night after the 'stilt' treatment was over.

She and I walked over arm in arm and I remember thinking we were like two winchers going to the picture house. I blushed and giggled when we sat down and Ina slipped her arm round my shoulders. I didn't know how to react – what to say. Was this what pals did? It felt lovely and cosy with her arm round me, her breast touching my side – she was so warm! I wanted to stay like that. We didn't hug or show affection in my family, so this was a new delicious experience for me. My pals and I had sniggered when we saw winchers sneaking into the bushes in the park or up 'back closes', but I did not know what they did there and I was not going to be laughed at by confessing this ignorance to my pals.

"We'll let on we're winchers," she whispered, crushing me to her with one hand and using the other to turn my face around, facing her. And then she kissed me on the lips.

'Quite nice,' I thought at first, until the smell of her made me pull away. It was a mixture of the cheap talcum powder with which she was always drenching herself and the smell of a wet-fish shop. It was awful! Why had I never noticed it before? She always sat really close when she was sitting at my bedside on visiting days, but all she had ever smelt of was talcum powder and lipstick.

It was the scent of sexual arousal, but I did not know that until I was much more grown-up and experienced.

When she was excited by the presence of the male porters, who were sometimes in the ward to shift furniture or clean windows, you could smell her a mile away, as the other women in the ward said, not caring whether she heard them or not. Many of them disliked her and were really cutting and cruel to her. It made no difference to her being nice to them. She just couldn't help herself. She had learned at an early age that sex was the way to get men to like her. Maybe she knew that it only made them despise her, but I honestly don't think she did.

I loved Ina, for her kindness and her way of making me laugh at her shocking stories, yet, little traitor that I was, I felt superior to her and, metaphorically, sneered behind my hand at her ignorance of almost everything. She had never read any of the books I had been brought up with, couldn't do even children's crosswords or answer the history or geography questions in the quiz books that Mrs God Bless You brought to us, or do arithmetic above the simplest of addition and subtraction (she told me that she had got the belt every day at school for getting her sums wrong), yet she made my time and that of most of the other women in the ward pass less darkly.

A few weeks after I came down from my perch I was just getting used to the new treatment that Dr Morton had promised me, and really enjoying my 'freedom', when Ina came into the ward after having been sent for by Sister. She was bouncing and beaming with excitement.

"Ah'm being moved to the convalescent ward," she shouted (shouting was forbidden) and did a little jig at the end of my bed. "Don't worry," she said, "ah'll be able to come and see you every day and we'll still go to the flicks together. Ah could be hame in a coupla months. Sister says the doctors want me to start building up my strength by going out on walks an' that." She came and gave me a hug. "And guess what? The best news of all – if ah keep doin' so well, ah'm tae get hame for a weekend – as long as ah've got somewhere to go." Her voice became less confident. "My Auntie Kate'll take me. She's got plenty o' room."

I put on a good act of being pleased for her, but my heart was black with jealousy and fear. I dreaded her leaving, but I could not spoil her happiness by being openly miserable, so I asked her what she would do on her weekend out.

Going to the dancing and getting a lumber played a big part in her plans, and her vivid description of what she intended to do with the lumber went a long way towards cheering me up – for a little while anyway.

The new treatment was not a pleasant experience, but I could thole it while I had my books, my visitors and my chats with Ina. Now that I was having one of my solaces taken from me the depression began to return, especially on treatment days, which were every Monday – in the morning.

The treatment was called artificial pneumothorax – AP for short – and involved collapsing the lung artificially by injecting air into the chest from under the arm. The actual needle was like a thick knitting needle, but the pain was bearable and you got used to it. What I hated was the choking feeling as the lung collapsed and curtailed the intake of oxygen to one lung. The idea was that the collapsed lung would be put out of use and so given a chance to heal. Once it had healed, the treatment would be stopped and the patient would have a strong healthy lung. It seemed to work for a lot of patients, so I was sure it would work for me.

The raised-bed treatment had been meant to rest and heal my left lung; the AP was targeted at the right. I was beginning to realise that Law Hospital was going to be my home for longer than the couple of weeks my dad had estimated.

It was like a neighbourhood street, with the fifteen beds on either side being our own little homes. Sister Taylor tried to limit what we kept on our lockers – a fruit bowl, a bottle of juice (provided by the NHS to some patients) and one or two photos – but few people stuck to her rules. Most of those with children had drawings done by their little ones as well as photos and other souvenirs. I had photos of my mum and dad, a diary sent by my sister, from London, a picture of Alan Ladd and some plastic word puzzles that Mrs Alexander had given me when she was leaving – oh, and a mirror, which I used a lot, to check whether I was looking better or not.

On visiting days – after the visitors had left – and in the evenings we visited one another's 'houses' to exchange gossip and share goodies brought by our visitors. Although I was depressed sometimes, after the failure of the 'stilt' treatment and news about Ina moving on, I think that I was basically a happy wee girl. I loved the linen sheets, the cosy red blankets, the stone hot-water bottles, having all the time in the world to read, going to see a film every week and, most of all, being the pet of everyone in the ward – patients, nurses, orderlies, Sister Taylor and even the doctors. I had never had so much love and attention in my fourteen years.

When I was eventually discharged, after just under four years, people would shake their heads and say, "Poor wee soul, losing four years of your life in that place." I went along with them and put on my most pathetic face, but I knew then, and I'm even more certain now, that those years were not lost. I learned much more from the time I spent in the world of Law Hospital, and getting to know about the lives of the women whom I met there, than I have ever learned since.

Ina was true to her promise and came to sit with me for a while every day, although sometimes she was restless to be with her new pals in the convalescent ward. I was not as upset as I might have been, for I soon had new pals of my own.

She came to see me on the Friday afternoon to tell me that she was going for her home weekend the next morning and promised to come on the Tuesday and tell me all her news.

What news! I couldn't sleep for nights for thinking about what she told me. It was more hair-raising than the Hank Janson books that were going the round of the ward, and which I had sneaked from one of the older women's beds when she wasn't looking.

More about Mr Janson later.

Ina had had to stay with her Auntie Kate, as her gran hadn't wanted the bother, and anyway she had a 'grotty auld tramp' staying with her. I envied her her exciting home life.

"Did you meet up with any of your boyfriends?" I asked (she had told me that she had hundreds of those). "Did you go to the dancing or the pictures? What did you wear? Was it good?"

She laughed and gave me a hug, and I noticed great black bruises on her arms and neck.

"God, what happened to you?" I asked. "You look as if you've been in a fight or something."

"My cousins did that," she said, pulling down her sleeves.

"They just got carried away, I guess. You know what fellas are like." She laughed again. "You'll find out soon enough, hen."

"What do you mean?" I asked. "What's that on your neck? It looks awful sore."

A shriek of laughter this time. "It's only a love bite. I'll give you one if you want. Jimmy (that's the oldest one) took me tae the pictures on Saturday – the matinee, ye ken – and then tae the pub. It was great fun, hen. Everybody wis buyin' me drink – gin an' orange – and we took fish and chips back tae ma Auntie Kate's. Oor Tommy was in – that's the youngest one. After we ate the chips, the two o' them had me on the couch. Ah wis too drunk tae stop them, even if ah hid wanted tae." She blushed and grinned. "Ah could hardly walk the next day – ah'm still sore, so ah am."

"You mean they forced you to let them have sex with you?" I could hardly get the words out for horror and embarrassment. "Did you not tell your auntie? Is it not rape [the first time I had ever said that word]? Did you not even scream?"

"Wheesht, hen. They've been daein' it since ah was a wean. They cannae help it. Men are like that. You'll know soon enough. It's as well tae let them have their way, so it is."

She went off back to her own ward after that. She looked sad. I think that I had put a damper on her weekend by my reaction to her story.

CHAPTER 6

FLORA

The first of my new pals was Flora McGregor – a sixteen-year-old from Islay, in the Inner Hebrides. I'm not sure why, but people were surprised to hear where she came from. Knowing no better, they assumed that TB would not affect people from a place that they associated with fresh air, sea breezes and outdoor pursuits like fishing, walking and curling. It was the filthy air of the cities that caused TB, wasn't it? How ignorant and wrong that assumption was! In my stay in Law Hospital I learned that many people from the Highlands and islands were victims. The reason there were more patients from the cities is simply that more people lived there.

Flora was one of the girls whose face and voice still are alive in my memory. To look at she reminded me of a picture that was in one of my books when I was a wee girl, of an elf sitting on a toadstool. Her whole face was pointed: chin, nose and even her hairline, which was shaped into a sharp widow's peak on her high pale forehead. Her eyes were very pale blue and seemed to be laughing at most people – not in a kind or friendly way. She did not appear to like the human race very much, and some of her contempt for many of the patients and staff, whom I had previously liked, infected me for a while.

When Margaret Harriday walked past the end of our beds (we were next to each other) carrying her china teacup and saucer, which she always washed herself, or wearing the huge metal curlers she put in most nights to maintain her 1940s hairstyle, Flora just had to look at me, with that scorn she had down to a T, for me to have to slide under the blankets to smother my laughter. I did not feel guilty about ridiculing a woman who had always been kind to me. I saw her through Flora's eyes and she was a figure of fun – inviting ridicule.

Sister Taylor also provided us with cruel amusement. She had a mannerism of pursing her lips if she disapproved of something – like an untidy bed or locker, or someone making a face as they swallowed their medicine – which Flora could imitate perfectly. She usually did this as Sister was trying to encourage me to take something for my 'own good', such as malt and cod-liver oil or cascara and liquid paraffin, when she would be facing me and her back would be to Flora, making her think that I was constipated or about to vomit – so dour and determined was my frown, to prevent myself from laughing. I did succumb once and spurted the disgusting mixture down Sister's starched front.

Another thing that amused Flora about Sister was the way in which she blushed and giggled when it was Dr Ballantine's turn to do the rounds, or if a male physio or radiologist visited the ward – in fact in the presence of anyone of the male sex. I had noticed this, but just put it down to being shy. In those days I was quite shy myself.

Flora knew exactly what was wrong with her: "She needs a man," she said. "I bet she's never even had her old fanny felt since her mother washed it."

After receiving this information, I blushed even redder than Sister every time it happened to her – which gave Flora a great laugh.

I didn't love Flora in the way I loved Ina, but she was somehow more exciting to be with (despite Ina's X-rated stories). I never knew what she would say next, or whom she would take down a peg, as she liked to say. Her cruel words were like arrows, and she always shot to kill, or at least inflict painful wounds.

Every Sunday afternoon during visiting hour there was a group of do-gooders, as Flora called them, who visited patients who for one reason or another did not have family or friends by their beds. Flora almost always fell into this category, so the Church Ladies always stopped by her bed with magazines, sweets, fruit and uplifting words of encouragement and cheer. Poor ladies, they did not expect to be met with such contemptuous hostility as that with which Flora greeted their Christian kindness!

I understood – or thought I did – why Flora hated these visits. She had explained to me why she seldom got visitors from home: her parents had been separated for years, and her mother lived in Paisley ("She works for some snotty rich family as housekeeper," she said.) and her father was a farmer at home on Islay. He flew down to Glasgow whenever he could, to visit her – which was about once a month, or less at the busy times on the farm. Her mother came even less, probably because Flora sat reading a book the whole time she was there, not even looking at the things she had brought, whereas when her father was there she giggled and chattered for the whole hour and held on to his hand when he was leaving as if she could not bear to let him go. I wondered why the parents had split up – judging by Flora's reactions, it must have been the mother's fault.

In my naive way I saw the situation as somehow romantic and hoped that someday Mr and Mrs McGregor would arrive at Flora's bed on the same day and be reunited, making Flora realise she loved them both and determined to get better so that she could go back to the farm with them. (My imagination balked at 'and live happily ever after', but the idea was at the back of my mind.)

Until that mythical day I continued to be shocked and delighted by my new pal's cruel treatment of almost everybody. She excelled herself with the Church Ladies. She really hated them. The more simperingly kind and concerned they were, the more she hated them.

The leader was like a model for knitwear out of *People's Friend*, which was very popular reading material with some of the women in the ward. (Mrs White brought a pile of copies every week.) She was always immaculate in her heather-mixture tweeds, one string of pearls, neatly bunned hairdo and pale-pink powder and lipstick. Her expression was one of constant smiling sympathy and understanding. A few times she spoke to me while I was waiting for my visitors to arrive, and she had the same effect on me as my first infant-school teacher had had – a kind of desperation to impress and ingratiate oneself.

The others – the numbers varied between four and six – were made in the same mould, with some minor variations, but Flora hated the leader most bitterly. Her name was Mrs White. Flora always referred to her as Mrs Shite, so while she was talking to me I avoided using her name just in case I had a slip of the tongue.

The others began to avoid Flora's bed, pretending that they were needed urgently elsewhere, but Mrs White – with great Christian fortitude – persisted. Flora always made a point of coughing disgustingly and using her sputum can during her visits.

One day I heard her asking the poor woman if she could "Bring me in some dirty books. The library here is rubbish."

Kind and Christian as she was, this request, nevertheless, succeeded in chasing Mrs White out of the ward – looking as if she was about to cry.

Flora laughed viciously and called after her, "Don't forget my books. Hank Janson's my favourite."

I would not say Hank Janson was my favourite writer, but his dirty paperbacks were part of the sex education I received in Law Hospital and I'm still grateful to him – whoever he was – for the pleasant times I spent curled under the blankets, sweating over his bad prose describing things going on between men and women that I could not have imagined without his help. Looking back, I realise his stories were pure schoolboy smut and would shock nobody nowadays, but they made it easier for us, who had to live apart from the outside world. They added a new dimension to lives bound by X-ray days, results days, visiting hours and Film Nights. I wonder if he was a real person. Some of the girls said he was a famous comedian writing under a pseudonym Others said he was actually a woman. I did not really care.

Flora took over from Ina in furthering my education, but her knowledge was gained from a different source – in a different world.

"I've never done it yet," she said. "You know – going the whole way wi' a lad. But I've got two lads waiting for me. We've done everything else. You know what I mean?"

My expression answered her question.

"Like kissing and touching everywhere. We've made each other come – do you know what that means?"

"Of course," I answered, willing her to tell me anyway.

Hank Janson had never written about that – whatever it was. Whom could I ask? I decided there was nobody – not even Ina.

Things were going really well for me at that time. I kept getting good reports from the Doctor.

I was gaining weight and Sister came beaming into the ward one day and told me, "Doctor has decided you can start going out for a short fifteen-minute walk in the afternoons – in clement weather, of course. What do you think of that?"

I thought it was the best news I had ever had in my life and was already picturing myself 'at the dancing' and going out wi' fellas almost before she had finished speaking.

"Of course you will be allowed up for visiting hours." Her face was glowing, and then she tried to be stern: "But you must take care. We don't want any setbacks, do we?"

With that she traipsed back out of the ward, her huge starched linen headress making her look like a sailing boat breasting the waves. At that moment I loved Sister Taylor.

I bounced on to Flora's bed, sure that she must have heard what Sister had said.

"What's wrong with you?" she snapped, moving away from me. "I'm busy writing to my dad."

He had not been able to visit her for three months.

"Did you not hear what she said to me?" I asked. "I'm to

be allowed up for visiting times and to go for a walk in the afternoons. Isn't it great!"

"It's only for fifteen minutes a day," she said, shifting further away from me and making a great show of having her pen poised to write in the pad on her poor bony knees. Like the unfeeling wee madam I was, I walked away down the ward to tell my news to people who would be happy for me – and stayed in a huff with Flora for over a week, telling myself that she was 'only jealous'. I should have understood. She was like the runt of the litter – left behind while her fitter, more attractive sisters moved on to a better future.

We were never as close friends after that. I could see that it upset her when I talked about the excitement of my walks and being able to go out with my visitors. But I couldn't talk about anything else! Apart from that, she'd had no visitors for months – she didn't count the Church Ladies and was more cutting to 'Mrs Shite' than ever – and her X-rays were showing little improvement. It went round the ward that her father had been sent for, and we thought the worst.

It was Nurse McKinnon, who told me that Flora was going home to Islay.

Even through my own selfish delight at 'getting better' I could see her becoming unhappier every day that went by without her getting a visitor.

"Surely her mum could come," I said to Ina one day as we sat on a seat just outside the ward. "She only lives in Paisley – that's not far away. Her dad's different. He'll be busy on the croft, I suppose."

"She wrote to her mother and told her not to come back," Ina said. "She told me. Ah think she's a cruel wee bitch at times."

"Well, I don't," I answered in my most self-righteous tone, drawing on my great experience of life at fourteen years old. "She left Flora and her wee brothers with their dad, so she doesn't deserve to see them now. That's what I think anyway."

"My ma left me wi' ma gran as soon as ah wis born." It was the first time I had seen Ina angry. "But ah wid still always want tae see her. You don't know how lucky you are tae have such a great family. No everybody's so lucky."

Nurse McKinnon came out of the French doors of the ward as we were speaking. She was smiling, as usual, but she looked sad.

"Right, you two," she called to us, "you've got company. Sister says Flora's to get some fresh air. You can cheer her up."

She turned back into the ward and returned, pushing the ward's ancient wooden wheelchair with Flora sitting in it nearly lost in pillows, and with a red blanket over her legs – although it was really warm in the sun.

She was smiling for the first time in weeks and suddenly I felt shy, as if she was a stranger. I could see Ina was looking embarrassed as well, and felt sorry for what I had been saying. Ina was right – what could I know about how people felt who were less lucky than me.

Soon the three of us were giggling, just like any other young girls enjoying the sunshine in each other's company. For an hour we forgot about the rotten worm inside us and talked about boys (Ina explained what 'Gama rouche' meant and nearly made me sick) and about what we would do when we got married, what kind of house we would have and how many kids, and whether we favoured big weddings or 'just running away'. Ina wanted loads of kids – a fitba' team. I wanted one of each – a boy and a girl. And Flora said she didn't ever want any.

"I never want to be anybody's mum," she said as a black cloud – as if on cue – covered the sun and made us shiver. "Get the nurse," she commanded Ina, "I've had enough fresh air. I want to go in."

That was my last conversation with her. Two weeks later screens were put around her bed in the early morning, and when they were removed she was sitting in the wheelchair wearing outdoor clothes and holding a little vanity case on her lap on top of the red blanket. Her cheeks were two little red blotches against the sick paleness of her skin and she was trying to wear her usual cynical smile in spite of the tears running down her cheeks and into her mouth. Nurse McKinnon was holding the back of the chair. She was wearing her cape and outdoor cap – looking like a Dutch doll, I thought – and carrying a small holdall. She wheeled Flora over to my bed and she handed me a box of sweets (I remembered her mother bringing them) and a pile of Hank Jansons.

'I'm going home to Islay," she said. "The doctors think I'll get better quicker at home. I'll write to you – mind and answer. All the best."

That was it. She did not do the 'leaving ritual': just a wave as she left the ward and that was the last we saw of her. Nurse McKinnon was going with her on the plane. We should have been happy for her going home, but most of us knew it was not because the doctors thought she would get better – just the opposite.

CHAPTER 7

PEN PALS

Any new craze or interest was a godsend in the ward, and there were plenty – from crocheting to writing to pen pals, to having a running competition, to seeing who could forecast the first record to be played on *Housewives' Choice* (there was a money prize for this). The best craze of all was having our photos taken by a professional photographer who was allowed into the ward on Friday evenings as long as Sister Taylor was not on duty.

He was the brother-in-law of one of the ward maids and had first appeared to take photos when a young bride had come to visit her mother just after the ceremony. I don't know which of the women first approached him to take other photos, but we were soon all eager to be 'models' and order photos to send to our relatives, friends and pen pals. Remember, cameras were still a bit of a novelty then and were usually only possessed by professionals. Having a photo taken was a big event – usually only experienced at weddings and other special occasions.

At first we were content with 'portraits' and posed groups, but as the bug bit some of us became more adventurous.

My brother-in-law Eric, who was in the RAF in Korea, had sent me a quilted bedjacket, red satin, with Chinese embroidery on it. I wore it with my black trousers for a picture for the family and (with much blushing and giggling) without the trousers for my pen pal – the borstal boy. (That led to a lot of trouble later on.) I didn't mind lending it to the other girls for their pictures. It was the most popular choice of costume, but after everyone who wanted had had a shot we were looking for new ideas.

Most of the older women were fed up with the craze and were beginning to grumble about the prices that they were charged for the prints; however, there was still a group of us who could not get enough of seeing ourselves in glossy print.

We were all sitting on Mary McKay's bed, on the Thursday night just before lights out, trying to come up with some ideas for Friday's 'performance'. There was Mary, Ina, Isabel Bain, Mary Kelly, Big Mary Hughes and myself and we were having a giggle about the mad suggestions being put forward.

It was Mary McKay who surprised us by saying, in her wee quiet boy's voice, "We could do a wedding party. It would be a great laugh – sure it would!"

Her face turned scarlet, expecting us all to laugh at her – and we did, rolling about the bed and screeching until the night nurse came and shouted at us to get into our own beds.

The idea seemed better the more we talked about it the next day on our 'time up' in the rec.

Mary McKay was popular from her arrival in the ward, partly because of the way she looked. There was something in her face that attracted the good feelings of nearly everyone to her. It was an expression that seemed to say you may as well like me, because I like you anyway – and that was how it was. She had dark, straight hair cut in a bob and those high cheekbones that were a legacy from the Polish ancestors which many people in Lanarkshire have. I suppose she might have been a beauty, but her body let her down. It was fine from the waist up, with nice rounded curves and straight shoulders, but her legs were stunted and bowed, making her walk like a caricature of a cowboy. Everyone felt sorry for her, but no one would ever hurt her by saying so. When my brothers or mother visited me she would remark enviously on how 'straight and slim' they were, depriving me of words in reply. I felt that there was nothing I could say without hurting her.

Mary decided that she would play the part of the minister in our pretend wedding photo. Next we had to decide on the bride and groom and their attendants and plan how to get costumes for them.

The other Mary – Mary Kelly – was selected as the bride. She was a tiny person (a pocket Venus was a popular description of her type in those days). Her rosy-complexioned face was framed by brown curls, which she did not have to create with the curlers most of the rest of us wore at bedtime. Her expression was almost nunlike in its innocence – contradicted by the dirty laugh of a barrow boy. She was engaged to be married, which was another reason for us choosing her as the bride, but her looks were the main decider.

Big Mary Hughes was to be the father of the bride, although Ina wondered how we would cover up her big 'bazookas'. Those two were always making remarks about one another's figures and their ability to 'get the men', but I always felt that Mary's remarks were more innocent than Ina's – as if she did not always understand the blue expressions and double meanings that occurred in Ina's every sentence. The idea of the wedding photo came up before that terrible day when Betty was brought back to the ward to die, so Mary was as loud and boisterous as ever and kept clutching the bride to her bosom and saying such things as "Come on, ma wee dochter, an' gie yer daddy a cuddle," much to Mary Kelly's embarrassment.

"Right," Mary McKay called us to order, really getting into her role as minister, "who's going to be the groom? Wee Jean's too young. It's between Ina and Isabel."

Ina jumped in: "Isabel's too wee and square-looking. The groom should be tall and slim – ah should be the groom." And then, leering wickedly: "Ah think Mary and ah will make a lovely couple."

She was trying to make Mary sit on her lap when one of the nurses came and told us it was time we were back in the ward. We quickly decided that I would be the bridesmaid and Isabel the best man, before obeying orders. That left only a mother of the bride to find, and none of us could think whom to ask.

Isabel Bain had not been a patient for very long, but she fitted in all right with our group, although she and the two Marys had been a bit wary of one another as she was a very vocal Protestant and Rangers supporter, from Cambuslang, whereas they were Tims, as she put it, from Glasgow and Celtic supporters. (Even in that place, it mattered to some people which side you were on in the argument which still divides a large area of Scotland.) Their jokes about Tims and Proddies were usually good-natured, yet you could sense the resentment underneath.

When the Friday night came for the wedding group to be posed we were all as nervous as if it had been the real thing. There was no mother of the bride. We couldn't agree whom to ask, so we made her a motherless child. The costumes were masterpieces of ingenuity: men's jackets had been brought in by Jimmy Hughes for the groom, best man and father of the bride; the bride's dress was pinned together from bed sheets (borrowed from the linen store), a piece of lace curtain and flowers removed from the vases in the ward. I wore a blue taffeta dress down to my feet, which Margaret Harriday lent me and pinned to fit my skinny figure, and a flower in my hair. The minister wore a black jacket borrowed from a porter and one of Jimmy's shirts on backwards. All of the 'men' had moustaches (black mascara) and the bride and I were made up like film stars. I was sick with excitement by the time the photographer arrived – more so than I was years later at my real wedding.

It did not take much to excite us in our unreal world, and everyone seemed to be infected. Just as if it had been a real bridal party being posed outside a real church, the whole ward formed an audience to see us being posed by the photographer, who looked as if he would die of embarrassment any minute. Others who wanted photos taken waited patiently, giving us priority, as if we really had just been through a ceremony which would start us off on a new life. I still get a lump in my throat when I think of our innocent pleasure in the imitation of an experience which many in that ward would never live to have in real life.

My family's reaction to the photo when they saw it varied. The boys laughed and looked embarrassed, asking me to point out the various members of the wedding party in the ward.

"The only nice-looking one is the bride." they agreed.

"The rest look as if they were oot fer their Hallowe'en," Robert added, and that was the extent of their interest.

My mother also looked embarrassed. "A lot of silly nonsense!" she said, shaking her head like an angry hen. "I'm surprised Sister Taylor allows it."

I explained that it happened when Sister was off duty. It would have been awful if she'd got into trouble with Matron because of us.

The strangest reaction was from Dad: he was furious.

"What the hell's going on in here?" he said. "Ah thought this was a place for ye to rest and get better, and here ye are posing wi' a crowd of queeries, dressed up like men and acting as if they were marryin' another woman. It's bloody sick! I've a good mind tae take ye out of here right now, so ah have."

I started to cry, not understanding why our innocent game was making him so angry. (He told me years later that he was always thinking that, because I was so young, "some lesbian would take advantage of you – these places were full of them".) He was so worried about my crying making me ill that he dropped the idea of making a fuss, just warning me to be careful whom I made friends with.

"I know about these things," he said. "It happens all the time in the army."

As I was in the dark about what 'these things' were, his warning was wasted, but I promised to tell him if any women 'approached' me, and that satisfied him, just a bit.

The photo of the wedding group was lost a long time ago, yet I can still picture us happily and innocently posing, not realising the message some people might have seen in it.

The photography craze became linked with another that was exciting many of the patients – writing to pen pals, which had some scary consequences.

The practice was really popular, even in the outside world, and there were many to choose from. Newspapers often had lists of servicemen serving abroad who were desperate for someone to write to them; women's magazines had a wider range, including foreign students, male and female. It was like the birth of the lonely hearts clubs and the dating sites on present-day computers. The letters we sent and received would start off innocently enough and then become more personal and in some cases outrageous. Even some of the married women had correspondents, and, apart from thinking up exciting lies to write, we had the hilarious, cruel pleasure of reading out the replies to the whole ward – or those who wanted to listen.

Margaret Harriday and some of the more strait-laced women were shocked and said that what we were doing was 'not nice'. We didn't care; the letters made us laugh, and laughter was a precious thing to us – no matter how cruel.

I started off with two pen pals, one a sailor in the Royal Navy, the other a German student. The first became more and more amorous with every letter – telling me things about his body parts that gave me nightmares – but he stopped writing after I sent a photo. Either I was not attractive enough to fit his fantasy or he guessed my age – I would never know. The German student petered out as our shortcomings in each other's languages became too much.

At this time Cathy Cummisky (another sad story) was in the next bed to me. Her friendship made me feel grown-up as she furthered my sex education with stories of her own experiences, which made my hair stand on end and my voice become hoarse. I was studying one of the women's magazines that Mrs God Bless You had left on my bed when Ina came bouncing into the ward and sat on my bed.

"What ye lookin' for?" she asked. "No another pen pal? Is two no enough?"

"I'm fed up with them," I answered. "I want somebody new – more my own age."

The sailor had claimed to be thirty-five and the student nineteen.

"Ah know just the lad for you!" Cathy called across.

"Who do you mean?" I asked, liking the sound of him already.

"He's my nephew."

Even better!

"And he's away frae hame as well – for a while. He gets really lonely. Ah'll give ye his address, but yer dad might no like ye writing to him."

Ina was panting with curiosity. "Why no?" she asked.

"He's a really good lad, but he got in wi' a bad crowd and got intae a wee bit o' trouble wi' the law – nothing serious, mind, but ye know whit thae auld judges are like [I had no idea]. They said they were makin' an example of him, so he got sent tae borstal for two years. It's a bloody shame."

My eyes were filling with tears when she had finished speaking. This was the ideal pen pal for me: a young boy locked away unjustly, lonely and definitely with no chance of being approved by my father.

"Ah'll write to him," I said, feeling like some kind of Florence Nightingale figure – full of love and self-sacrifice.

Cathy rummaged about in her locker and brought out a tiny brown envelope, from which she took out two very thin sheets of paper which she then returned to the locker.

"I'll write the address on here," she said. "He wrote to me last week. Maybe ye'd better not tell yer da, eh?"

Ina flounced away in a jealous huff. She didn't like my being friendly with Cathy, whom she considered 'a right scruff '.

I wrote right away. I blushed for a long time whenever I recalled that first letter. I bet the other borstal boys loved it. My 'romance' with Frankie Coulter had begun and would hover about like a virus waiting to strike for a long time afterwards.

Sister Taylor frowned and put on her best pout as she scrutinised the envelope containing his reply before handing it to me. No wonder! It was smaller than any envelope I was used to, it was brown and looked a bit grubby, and it had an official frank on it instead of a stamp. I felt as if I was receiving something illegal and could hardly wait to open it. I didn't want to open it in public. I had no intention of reading it out – not in front of Cathy, so I hurried off to the toilets, holding it in my dressing-gown pocket.

'Dear Jean,' it began. 'Ma Anty Cathy says yoor a reely good lookin' bit o' stuff [I cringed at the spelling mistakes], she sez ye want a pen pal, well sody ah. Ah huv tae be onest. A' the lads in here talk aboot is lasses an' gettin' thur candy, bit ah'm no like that, Jean. Ah wid like a good [there was a blacked-out word here], bit ah wid want tae get tae no the lassie furst. Ah wid want ye tae be ma girlfriend. Rite back an' tell me what ye think, an' send a photie. Yours truly, Frankie. xxxxxxx

The letter gave me the strangest mixture of feelings: I despised the bad spelling, yet the roughness of the tone of the letter excited me, as did wondering what the blacked-out word was. (Whom could I ask?) I felt really daring getting a letter from someone who had been in trouble, and I was torn between being the really good woman who would save him from the bad crowd and turn him into someone like my dad, or joining up with the bad crowd and being the kind of woman that strutted through the pages of Hank Janson. I decided to answer his letter anyway and send a photo and see what happened after that.

I let Cathy see the letter. She told me what the blacked-out word would be and explained that their letters were censored, which thrilled me no end. When I told Ina, she told me to ask him if he had any pals who would like a letter from her.

The next thing was to pick a photo to send. I didn't want to put him off by looking too young or in bed like an invalid, so I decided on the one I had had taken in my Chinese jacket – without my trousers on – looking like a principal boy (I thought), and Cathy and Ina agreed that it was 'a smashin' photo' and said he would probably put it up on his wall, which made me feel like Betty Grable.

At first I really looked forward to getting the funny little brown envelopes and seeing the huffy look on Sister Taylor's face as she handed them to me. Frankie's spelling never got any better, but his imagination was obviously in good fettle as he described the 'grate times weel huv when ah get oot o' here, doll'. The blacked-out words took up a big part of the letters and it was not hard – even for me – to guess that most of them had to do with sex. It was the bad spelling that finally put me off – I was developing quite a strong streak of snobbishness in my nature, probably due to having discovered Jane Austen.

I wanted to stop writing to him, but I couldn't think of hurting Cathy, so I kept going for a while longer, until Cathy told me she was going home – signing herself out, just as Teresa Gray had done and for much the same reason: on the orders of her man. It made me really sad to know that she was going. I was worried for her after the stories she had told me about this bloke that she was willing to risk her survival for.

They had grown up in the same street in the Cowcaddens area of Glasgow.

"He was ma big brother's best pal," she said. "He never really looked at me, although he was always in an' out of our house, an' ah use tae make eyes at him like a wee slut. He'd pu' ma hair and tickle me under the oxters 'til ah nearly wet maself laughin', but it wisnae 'til ah wis fifteen that he started lookin' at me wi' that look that men get in their eye – ye know whit ah mean?"

I nodded knowingly, from my great experience of men, and she laughed and gave me a cuddle.

"It wis great at first," she went on. "He had joined the navy – you should have seen him in his bell-bottoms, wi' his hat sittin' on the side of his head like a pea on a dumplin' – and he asked ma da if we could get engaged. Da wisnae bothered – he was glad to get rid of me. He knew ah wid get nicket sooner or later. This way he could get me aff his hands. So we got married as soon as ah turned sixteen, and we got a wee single-end in Gallowgate. It wis great at first. He was stationed in Dunoon and came hame every weekend. Then we had our first big fight, because ah went tae the pictures wi' ma pal when he was away. He slapped me an' ah ran round tae ma da's, but he told me ah had made ma bed an' wid have tae lie in it. He walked in an' told me tae get ma coat, an' ah did. Before we reached our close he pulled me intae a back court, an' ah suppose people would say he raped me. That was when ah fell pregnant wi' ma wee Babs. He was really kind an' nice tae me for a while after that, so he wis."

My stomach was churning with the horror and excitement I felt in hearing her story. This was better than anything Hank Janson had ever written.

"Did you not report him – to the police, I mean?" I asked hoarsely.

"Ye cannae report yer man fer rape, hen," she said. "It's his right, in law."

For years I believed this was true. A lot of the 'education' I got from the other patients was like that. I found out that so much of it was wrong, but they had lived their poor lives thinking it was the way things had to be. Ina and Cathy believed that men had the right to do what they wanted with them.

The back-court rape was not the worst of Cathy's stories. Her next one gave me nightmares and nearly put me off all men for life.

"After ah had wee Babs," she said, "we were gettin' on great and when she was only a year old ah fell pregnant wi' oor wee Tommy. Then it a' went wrong. Hugh [Cathy's man] was posted down tae England – tae Plymouth – an' ah wis left on ma oan wi' jist the wean fer company. But ah didnae mind. Ah wis really happy, an' he said ah could go down an' visit him. He said it wid be like bein' on honeymoon and his mother wid watch wee Babs an' let me go maself. Ah wis that excited!"

Ina and I were about swooning with excitement and Ina's smell was overpowering. I hoped I would never smell like that.

"Ah was a bit sick on the train going down, bein' just a month gone, but ah didnae care. Ah thought he would be there to meet me, but he wasn't, so ah asked directions tae the base and started walking. Ma case was gettin' heavier by the minute. When a fella in a Jeep stopped an' offered me a lift, ah couldnae jump in quick enough."

She told us how he had 'seemed really nice and friendly' and told her how much he missed home and his girlfriend. When he turned off the road, she thought at first that they were turning into a driveway that would be the entrance to the base, then she realised that they were driving into an open field and asked him what was going on. He just laughed, jumped out and opened the passenger door.

"He was that strong," she said, "that he just lifted me out and carried me further into the field. There were haystacks and he just threw me down and was on top of me before ah could even yell. When ah did let out a scream, he just laughed an' telt me naebody could hear me."

"Did he rape ye?" Ina gasped.

Cathy took a minute or two to answer as if she was thinking what to say: "Ah let him, so ah don't suppose it wis rape, although ah didnae want him to dae it. Ah wis scared he would hurt me and the wee wean inside me. Ah just lay there an' let him get on wi' it – gruntin' like a pig. He helped me intae the Jeep when he wis finished, and a wee bit along the road he dropped me off at the gates tae the barracks an' a soldier took me tae the married quarters where ma Hugh wis waitin' for me."

Her voice shook as she went on with the story. I think she was sorry she had started it – telling us how she broke down when they were in bed and told him what had happened. He was mad at the man who had done it to her, but he was madder at her for 'letting him'. When she said that she wanted to report the attack and that she could identify her attacker, she thought he was going to strike her he was so mad with rage.

"He told me to keep my mouth shut," she explained. "He said he would be the laughin' stock wi' a' his mates if it got round that his wife was a hoor that let herself be picked up by any sojer that wis nice tae her. Ah knew that was what he had made up his mind tae think so ah didnae argue. It's always better tae keep the peace wi' ma Hugh, even when ye know he's wrong."

Under the tuition of Ina and Cathy I was losing the romantic little-girl notions about love that my diet of Jane Austen had nurtured (spoiled a bit by Hank Janson's jaundiced view), and I was getting desperate to find a way out of my long-distance romance with 'oor Frankie' when Cathy popped her head round the screens, which the nurses had put round her bed, just after visiting time one Saturday. I could see that she had been crying and she looked really ill, her lovely Garbo-like face scrunched up with sadness.

"Hugh's come fer me, pal," she said, and I thought of an executioner waiting to take her to the gallows. "His ma cannae cope wi' the weans, an' ah can get treatment just as well outside.

Ah'll write tae ye, an' we'll meet up when ye get out. Who knows, mebbe we'll be related some day, eh?"

The best part of me was heartbroken to lose my pal, yet there was a part that was glad of the opportunity to get out of writing to her nephew without having to tell her to her face – wee coward!

She had taken my hand to wish each other 'all the best', as was the custom when anyone was leaving, when a big hand was thrust round the screen and she was pulled out of sight to the sound of "Come on, you! Ah want tae get tae the match, an' we've tae get the weans frae ma ma's."

That was the last I saw of Cathy. We heard from Mrs God Bless You that she had been taken into another hospital in Glasgow, just a few weeks after she left Law Hospital, and died less than a month after. Her weans had been taken into a home in Dunoon and that's how she had heard about it. She visited the children there and took their news back to their mothers in various sanatoria. Cummisky is not a name you hear every day, and when she heard it she remembered Cathy and heard about her sad end from the matron of the home.

It was not the last I heard of 'oor Frankie', even though our correspondence came to an end when Cathy left. The wee brown envelopes put in a reappearance a couple of years later – to my horror.

CHAPTER 8

GOODBYES

One of the worst goodbyes was that to Cathy Brannigan, and it was not really a goodbye, in the sense that the words were never spoken. Everyone knew she was dying from the day she was moved into the cubicle after her spectacular haemorrhage. If we had not guessed from that, we could hear the pain of her dying, night and day. It was like listening to a wounded animal caught in a trap. The other deaths in the ward had left me almost unaffected. Although I had known those who died, their deaths were made anonymous by the way in which they were spirited out of the ward, with only the sound of the metal wheels of the mortuary trolley to signal their passing, behind the wall of protective screens, which made a tunnel to save us distress.

Cathy's death was public in that we all heard it happening.

"It's the bedsores," the night nurse – Nurse Gemmel – told us. "Poor soul, nothing can help her. Her bones are just jutting out of what's left of her skin. There's only so much morphine we can give her without killing her. It'll no be long now, I hope."

Naive as I was, I was shocked at a nurse admitting she could not help her patient and wishing she would die soon, but I found that everyone else felt the same as she did.

"It's the awful greetin'," Big Mary said. "Ah wish they could just put her to sleep and give her peace. Ah shouldnae say that, as a Catholic, but this is too cruel. The poor lassie doesnae deserve this. Naebody does."

It was a Saturday morning when I saw the last of Cathy. Nurse McKinnon had been washing my hair and setting it, ready for visiting time. We were walking past the cubicle – Cathy had hardly made a sound the previous night – when Sister Taylor came out with her finger to her lips. She pointed to the duty room and Nurse McKinnon went to follow her in, leaving me to make my way back into the ward. Sister shook her head and indicated that she wanted me to come into the office too. I began to think that something bad must have happened at home and Sister was about to break some terrible news to me. She closed the door quietly and I noticed that there were tears trapped behind her glasses.

"I'm going to ask you to do something, Jean", she said, "that will be very upsetting."

Nurse McKinnon put her arm through mine and gave it a squeeze.

"You can say no. Nobody would blame you if you do. It's Cathy. She heard your voice when you passed her room a little while ago and she perked up a bit – we thought she was sleeping. She's asking to see you."

Nurse McKinnon spoke before I could answer: "No, Sister! It would be too upsetting. A wee girl shouldn't see Cathy the way she is now. It would be too much to take."

"I don't think she will last the day," Sister said, "and she is so fond of Jean. Let her decide."

I thought guiltily of all the times I had laughed at Cathy and spurned her kindnesses to me, and, growing up a little bit more, I said, "Of course I'll go in and see her if it will make her feel better."

The blinds were drawn, so the figure in the bed seemed to be spotlighted by the shaded light above her bed. I didn't recognise her. She had turned into a shrunken 100-year-old witch. Her face was half the size it had been, which made her nose look like a huge beak, and her eyes were sunken so far into her head they were almost invisible; her hair was just a few poor lank strands combed across her skull, held in place by a giant kirby grip; her exposed ears looked as if someone had made them out of rice paper as part of a grotesque Hallowe'en mask. I took one look at this horror and tried to focus my eyes elsewhere. They alighted on her hands, the sight of which made me shiver. She was propped up straight and her hands rested on a kind of mountain of bedclothes. (I found out later they were supported by a wire cage to protect her legs from their touch.) They did not look like a human's hands, or those of any animal I had ever seen. The fingers were indistinguishable in a swollen mass of purple-coloured dough. She held one of them out to me.

"I wanted you to see my birthday present," she said, and I saw, embedded in the 'dough', a gold watch in the style referred to as a cocktail watch. "Come over a bit and see it. I won't bite you, you know."

The sound she made at her little joke wasn't a cackle or a laugh; it was a rattle as if her insides were breaking up and it led to a cough, which made me run from the room, saying as I went, "I'll come back tomorrow and see you, Cathy."

I could not have gone back, not for anything, but it did not matter because she died that night, and when I peeped into the cubicle the bed was stripped as if she had never been there. I hadn't even heard the clatter of the trolley taking her away. After I had left the cubicle, I had curled up in bed under the blankets until Mum and Dad arrived at visiting hour. I couldn't tell them about what I had seen – I couldn't talk about it to anyone – so I listened to talk about the family and neighbours and contributed stories about the other patients and what I had been reading. Mum had brought a box of cakes out of Peacocks, the bakery, and urged me to try them, but I said I would keep them for later. I thought that I would never be able to put food into my mouth again without vomiting.

Strangely, I slept really soundly, without dreaming of that shrunken head and the deformed paws, but it was my last nightmare-less sleep for a long time.

Nurse McKinnon told me that Cathy had died on her twenty-fourth birthday. I had always thought of her as ancient.

Until Cathy's death, none of the horror of the experience which I was sharing with my ward-mates had really touched me. I was more concerned with doing my hair in different styles, wearing make-up for the first time, and talking about the sex I was learning about from books and my pals' stories. Visiting days were the highlights of my life. I had no worries really, except occasionally to wonder when I would leave and take up a normal life. The friends who had left – and stories which sometimes reached us of their sad endings – did not remain in my memory for long. I remember them more vividly now. The sound of the mortuary trolley on its noisy but invisible journey had caused a slight shiver in my heart before I went back to my book, or my dreams, but before seeing that wizened wreck that Cathy had become it had meant nothing to me. Now I could not get the thought out of my mind that maybe my time was coming to be carted out on that rattling trolley.

We seldom talked about death; I suppose it was too much of a reality to be allowed into the unreal world in which we lived. The older women did – in soft, sad voices, hushed when any of us younger people came close enough to hear. I wanted to talk about Cathy, but I couldn't – not to my pals, or even Nurse McKinnon – so it festered like a running sore in my mind and, for a while, took all the joy out of my life. I wished Sister Taylor had never taken me into that room.

I was now allowed to go for a fifteen-minute walk in the grounds or sit in the rec with the other up-patients if the weather was inclement, as Sister Taylor said. I should have been happy as everyone saw this as a sign that I was getting better. To keep Cathy out of my mind I laughed a lot and talked excitedly on my walks – usually with Ina and Big Mary – and shouted greetings to any men who came in sight. I was like someone whistling in the dark to scare off ghosts, and it was beginning to work until one sunny day when we had just returned to the ward for 'rest hour'. I was laughing at something Ina had said or done when the laugh turned to a strange gurgling in my chest and a large blob of bright-red blood shot from my mouth on to the white linen sheet. I remember thinking it was like the ruby pendant Margaret Harriday sometimes wore.

Then Big Mary went rushing from my bedside, calling in a

terrified voice, "Nurse! Nurse! Wee Jean's sick! Come quick! Oh God!"

The coffee-coloured screens that I had watched being drawn around the beds of many of my fellow patients before they were taken away to the side room to die, or until the mortuary trolley rattled down the corridor and took them away, were now drawn, like a cloud shutting out the sun, around my bed. Sister Taylor and skinny little Nurse Brown – who rumour said was a drug addict – came bustling in and built pillows behind my back so that I was sitting straight up, before Sister took a syringe from the medicine tray which she had placed on my locker when she came in.

"I want you to keep very still and calm, Jean," she said in a commanding voice that reminded me of a very strict primary teacher I once had.

I nodded, feeling my terror die down a bit with the knowledge that Sister would make everything all right again.

"That's right," she said, "don't talk. I'm just going to give you this little injection that will stop the blood. Dr Morton is on her way. She told me to tell you to be a brave girl and not to worry."

I suddenly felt that I loved this shy starchy old maid and I disobeyed her orders to tell her so, in a very sleepy voice, as the dose of morphine began to take effect: "I love you, Sister Taylor," I muttered, and was rewarded with one of her most spectacular blushes as I drifted off.

The slight haemorrhage I had suffered was more dramatic than serious, but I was made a bed-patient once again for a couple of weeks. I was allowed up again after the results of an X-ray showed that there was no further damage to my lungs. The Doctor said that the blood was probably from scars that had healed and it was 'better out than in' and I believed her, but, looking back, I think that this must have been when it was decided that the drugs, raised-bed treatment and artificial pneumothorax were not going to be enough to see the end of the disease and surgery would be required, although no one said that until a while afterwards.

As the treatment discovered by Dr C was proving to be the answer to finding a cure for TB, patients were admitted and left in a much shorter time and friendships were ever more fleeting. Flora was gone, and Nurse McKinnon got a letter telling her that she had died just two months after she was home in Islay; Big Mary Hughes was discharged as cured and was now helping Jimmy in visiting the last of their wee sisters, who was in Mearnskirk and responding to treatment; Ina was discharged and pregnant within three months; Mary McKay was discharged, 'cured', as were many others of my friends who had been admitted after me. I tried not to be downhearted about this, but I was. The only one of the patients who had been there when I arrived was Margaret Harriday, looking more and more like an ageing forties film star and being told after every X-ray that she was 'making good progress' and just needed to be 'a bit stronger' before she got home.

I asked Dr Morton why I could not be sent to the convalescent ward now that I was an up-patient, and she said that she would talk to her husband, Dr Ballantine, about it, but I was sure that she was just putting me off.

I began a campaign of huffing and moaning to anyone who would listen. I cried to my father that I wanted to go home and refused to eat the dinners Mum brought me on a Sunday. None of this worked, so I tried a new tack – rebelling.

There was a new patient in the ward who really interested me. Her name was Hetty Aiken. She was quite an ugly-looking woman really by today's standards. She had smooth, very white skin and dark hair streaked with grey, and maybe would have been attractive but for her enormous horse-like buck teeth, which she showed a lot of because she was always laughing or smiling. The bane of Sister Taylor's life, she made her blush every day, yet she seemed to kind of like it, like the girl who pretends to be shocked at men's suggestive remarks while enjoying them.

I loved Hetty. She was married with three children, who were being cared for by their father and her mother, and another one was on the way.

"Naebody's pittin' ma weans intae a home," she said often enough to offend the other mothers in the ward, who had no choice in the matter.

Many of them didn't like her and did not try to hide it. She sang without fuss, when threatened with Malcolm talcumming, a dirty song about the island of Gibraltar standing on a rock and 'every man that goes there has to show his cock'. There were much worse things said in the ward, but this seemed to affront everybody – maybe because it was sung.

I was fascinated by her wee bundle, as she referred to the expected baby, and her openness about discussing it and what had led up to it being there. When my eldest sister had been pregnant any conversations regarding her condition were spoken in whispers and stopped immediately if my brothers or I were in earshot. Not so with Hetty, who took Ina, Big Mary and me through every symptom and even told us about the conception – which cleared up the few remaining gaps in my sex education.

"Ah told ma Tommy ah wis havin' nae mair," she said, "but the auld devil got me drunk on oor anniversary, and ah wis that randy ah forgot a' aboot bein' careful. Still, it's as easy tae feed four as three, an ah've got a guid man."

I was not quite sure what she meant about being careful, but she and Ina soon explained about French letters and other things that made me feel quite sick. My romantic notions were once more taking a bashing.

The other thing I loved about Hetty was the way she didn't care what she said, even to the doctors, and how she broke all the rules apart from the one that barred smoking. She was supposed to have only three hours 'up time', but she hardly ever seemed to be in her own bed, sometimes even after lights-out. She joked with even the strictest nurses – even Nurse Gemmel, of whom everyone else was terrified – and stayed outside the ward much longer than the half-hour that she was allowed. It was this that eventually led to her getting into real trouble with the doctors and being sent home.

She would probably have got away with a telling-off from the Doctor, but she included me and Ina in her escapade and Dad was furious with the hospital for 'not keeping an eye' on me and letting me be 'led astray' by a stupid woman. Although she had not made us do anything we didn't want to do, she was older and should have known better, according to everyone but us. I tried to make Dad see that I had been as much to blame as her, but he was having none of it. Looking back, I think his fear of lesbians and corruption was at the root of his extreme reaction, and poor Hetty was the scapegoat the doctors used to placate him. He could be very scary when he was angry.

It was such a simple, harmless thing we did (although now I can understand the panic it caused). The three of us were having our afternoon stroll in the grounds and decided to go to the little shop-cum-café just outside the gate for a cup of tea and a bun. It was Ina that planted the idea of going further, although I don't think she meant it seriously.

"Sure, it would be great to just jump on a bus and spend a wee while in Wishaw an' see the shops," she said. "Ah'm bored wi' this wee café. Ye never see anybody but patients like us."

"We could easily slip away for a wee while," Hetty said, showing her big wet teeth in a wicked grin. "We could get the next bus back an' be in the ward before teatime. Ah would like to buy a present for my wee Suzy. It's her birthday next week an' ye cannae trust a man tae pick a present for a wee lassie."

"Come on, we'll ask Geordie [the shop owner] when the next bus is," said Ina, and then, pointing along the road: "Look – here's one coming now. Let's get it!"

I felt as though everyone on the bus knew we were 'escapees', but Hetty's and Ina's excitement infected me and I felt like one of the Famous Five off on 'an amazing adventure'. We had no thought of being found out or what would happen if we were. Oh, that taste of freedom was intoxicating. I could not stop giggling. It was over two years since I had been outside and every shop was exciting and glamorous to me, yet I was afraid too – afraid of being surrounded by so many hurrying people, afraid of street noises which I had never noticed before.

Hetty took ages – it seemed to me – to choose a white cardigan and matching lacy white socks for her wee girl. Ina went into Boots and bought a bright-orange lipstick and I couldn't tear myself away from a big bookshop, where I bought a couple of film magazines and a 'true love story' book.

We then bought a bag of chips each and sat in a little park just by the bus stop to eat them, feeling like weans plunking school.

We had finished the chips and a cold wind was getting up when it dawned on us that the next bus back was not coming as soon as we had thought. Ina went up to a man standing at the bus stop.

"When's the next bus back to Law Hospital, mister?" she asked.

He looked at his watch. "There's one no long away. It'll be another half an hour," he answered, hardly looking up from his paper. "They don't a' stop at Law – only at visiting times," he added, and we knew we were bound to be missed at teatime. It was five o'clock already, and not a visiting night.

Eventually we reached the ward at six o'clock. Hetty had had to persuade the bus conductor that she was about to spew all over his bus if he didn't stop at the hospital gates, and then we had a freezing walk up the avenue. My teeth would not stop chittering and I felt like crying. The other two kept up a show of bravado, even when Sister Taylor met us at the duty-room door and told us that Dr Ballantyne and Dr Morton were inside and wanted an explanation for our absence.

She held me back and called to Nurse McKinnon to "Put this one straight into her bed with a hot-water bottle before she gets pneumonia. God knows what your dad will say about this, young lady."

I wanted to say that there was no need to tell him, but I was shivering too much to get the words out.

He knew all right! Sister Taylor had phoned his work. We did not have a phone at home. Few working-class families did in the 1950s. Dr Morton had told her to do so when we had not been in for our tea. I was a minor and they were responsible for me – this had not occurred to Hetty when she had let me be involved in the adventure.

Big Mary emerged from the duty room first and rushed past my bed in tears.

"They're sending Hetty away!" she called out before

throwing herself on to her bed and pulling the blankets over her head.

Most of the women were shocked, with quite a few voicing the thought 'It serves her right – taking two young lassies out like that – daft bitch!'

I sat up and stared at the entrance to the ward, dreading my friend entering. Where could they send her? What about her treatment? What would her man say? And would they send me away too?

Her face was whiter than it had ever been and her attempt at giving me a flash of her big teeth did not come off. She took a small suitcase from the foot of her wardrobe and started packing it with the photos and things from her locker. Coming to my bed, she handed me one of the photos of her and her daughters.

"Take this, hen," she said, "as a memory of your bad Auntie Hetty. Ah'm sorry if you get intae trouble. Ah told them it's a' ma blame. Ah should have known no tae rely on these stupid buses."

The tears were running down into her mouth as she gave me a hug and a wet kiss on my cheek and turned to leave the ward with a cheeky wave to the other patients.

That was the last I saw of her. She did write once to tell me that she had been transferred to another hospital, closer to where she lived – in Helensburgh – and was doing fine, looking forward to her 'wee bundle' arriving. I had been given strict orders by Dad and Dr Morton not to contact her, so I didn't, although I thought about her often for a long time afterwards.

I continued my rebellion, turning away my food, speaking only when I was forced to – like the silly wee girl I was. I nursed a grudge against the world – particularly the doctors and my dad, whom I blamed for Hetty being sent away. I remember how I hurt him and blush at the memory.

Our family never showed physical affection to one another, apart from Dad, who always hugged me and gave me a kiss on the lips when he arrived at visiting time and when he left. I think he wanted to show that he was not afraid of catching anything, and also to show his love for me. I was too ungrateful and self-centred to understand that then, so I did a truly heartless thing: when he bent to kiss me on the first visit after the Hetty incident I turned my face away. The look on his face was awful. I could not have done worse if I had slapped him – but I did not care. I wanted to hurt everyone who had sent Hetty away. There was no one as much fun as her in the ward now, and Big Mary had been transferred to the convalescent ward. Self-pityingly I was convinced that they were taking all my friends away from me.

My rebellion was soon over, due to the news Sister Taylor delivered one Friday morning. She was fairly glowing when she hurried up to my bed, after Dr Morton had been on her rounds and I had ignored her usual friendly words to me.

"Well, young lady," she said, "get up and get dressed [for a minute I thought that I was being sent home]. Nurse McKinnon will help you to get your belongings. You're going to the convalescent ward. Dr Morton says you're ready for it – as long as you behave. No more running away!"

She actually giggled when she said this, before hurrying off down the ward, passing Ina, who was coming to help me empty my locker and load up the tea trolley to transport my stuff to Ward 26 – the convalescent ward – one step away from going home.

I spent a really happy three months there, but it did not lead to going home – not for a long time anyway. A lot would happen before that.

CHAPTER 9

THE CONVALESCENT WARD

I felt really happy there. The weather was warm, so we spent most days sitting out in stripy deckchairs, which the ward maids put out in the morning and stored away at night. It was just like being on holiday – even the smell was different. We were always aware that the disinfectant smell of the sick ward, as I now referred to my former 'home', was a layer covering the stench of bedpans and sick bowls. I had become used to it and it hadn't really bothered me, but I did appreciate the mixture of talcum powder, perfume and face-powder smells that pervaded Ward 26. It made me feel so feminine and grown-up.

There were only a few of the patients who had been in Ward 28 with me, so I had a lot of new people to get to know. I hardly thought of Margaret Harriday – still waiting to be 'strong enough' to go home. My new ward-mates were much more fun and they mostly treated me as a grown-up, although I still enjoyed the status of ward pet. They hardly talked about the illness, taking X-rays and results days in their stride – just steps to going home or being transferred to Hairmyres Hospital, where lung surgery was carried out (another step nearer home). The talk was mostly about sex, make-up, fashion and the latest 'true romances', and they did not become silent or hush one another when I was in earshot. I had no more desire to be in the huff or rebel. I knew it was only a matter of time until I would be told that I was going home, and this was a great place to wait for that day.

I do remember many of the girls who were there, but only as kind of snapshots in my life. There were no long-term relationships formed, apart from that with Ina. Nevertheless some of them made a lasting impression on me and I can still flick through my memory and see their faces and hear their voices.

There was a woman called Marion who had the yellowest dyed hair I had ever seen. She used to make us blush and laugh with her descriptions of how desperate she was for a man.

"Ah don't care whether he's wee and fat or tall and skinny," she would say, "as long as he's got the right bits in the right places and knows how tae use them."

She was always having 'wet dreams' about any man who came into her sights – even newsmen on the television. Her favourite of these was a man called McDonald Hobley, whom Ina and I thought looked like a walking skeleton. She only ever had one visitor – her sister, who had yellow hair like hers and was equally manless.

"It's no for the want o' trying," Marion would tell us. "We were never out of the Barrowland, an' we're baith braw dancers. We were never short o' lumbers, but it never came to anything."

There was no Malcolm talcumming in the convalescent ward, but we still had sing-songs. Marion's party piece was "Oh dear me, whit will ah dae if ah die an auld maid in a garret!"

Ina said more than once that she was 'probably queer', but I did not believe that, mainly because I did not want to.

Another of my snapshot memories is of a girl called Clare Meichan. She had nothing in common with Marion, although she was friendly towards everyone and laughed, as if at a silly little girl, at Marion's crush on McDonald Hobley, whom she described as a 'death's head with a nice smile'. I thought this description was so witty and funny. I wished that I had said it. Still, Clare was a schoolteacher, so she was expected to be clever.

She occupied the very last bed at the top end of the ward, which meant that she had more 'wall space' than me. I was in the next bed to hers and she won me over completely by letting me put up pin-ups of my favourite film stars – John Derek and Rory Calhoun – on her wall. I used to gaze at them before lights out so that I could plan the dreams I intended to have about one or other of them. These dreams were as erotic, romantic and exciting as my reading of Hank Janson and the sex education I had received from fellow patients could make them. I never confided in Clare about them. I did not want her to smile at me with the same expression that she wore with Marion. I wanted her to think well of me, so I asked her advice about what books to read so that I could 'take up my education' when I got home.

Of course Jane Austen was at the top of her list, and she was really impressed that I had already read *Pride and Prejudice*. Next was Charles Dickens – also no stranger to me, thanks to my dad – but she told me that there were other authors, like Agatha Christie and Denise Robbins, who wrote whodunnits which were clever and enjoyable to read, although not exactly classics.

"Reading's meant to be enjoyable as well as educational," she often said, "but you waste your intelligence and your time if you read the rubbish some of these women read. They do not know any better, but you do." I suppose, looking back, she was a bit pompous and an intellectual snob; but so was I and she did give me my love of a good whodunnit, which has got me through many difficult times.

Clare was only twenty-four and in appearance entirely different from Marion, Ina or any of my other friends. She was tall and walked with her head held high, as if she was very conscious of her height and proud of it. Her hair was black and dry, without the gloss you usually associate with black hair. She hated its dull dryness and was always trying new shampoos and treatments for it. That and her height seemed to be her only vanities. She never wore make-up – not even lipstick – which I thought was very odd, as did my friends, who spent hours doing up their faces and bodies.

I learned as much from Clare, however, as I did from my other 'teachers'. She taught me that one bath a week was not enough if one wanted to be 'nice' in the presence of others.

"If you can't get a proper bath every day," she said, "at least have an all-over body wash when you get up in the morning and wash your hair as often as you can."

I thought that that was probably why hers was so dry – she was always washing it and spent most of her time with a towel around her head like some female Sikh – but I didn't voice this opinion. I was never cheeky to her as I was to the other 'older' women. It was she who showed me that I was often really hurtful when I thought I was just being smart. I was forever making remarks about the few fat women in the ward, and I called anyone whom I considered old an 'old fossil'. Clare convinced me that was the wrong way to behave. No one had ever pointed this out to me before. In fact my 'pals' encouraged me and called me a 'great laugh'.

It wasn't that she was in any way an old fossil. She had a really good sense of humour and had us in stitches sometimes with her stories of the time she had spent teaching in a big school in London. She could do accents like an accomplished actress, changing from the Cockney of the pupils to the upper class of the head teacher in a breath. I thought that she was probably upper class, being a teacher, and I wanted to be like her. Ina and Big Mary seemed very common to me now.

I asked her once how she had caught TB, thinking it was probably from some of the lower-class children she had taught. She explained sadly that she had looked after her sister when she had caught it from her husband, whom she had nursed on his deathbed. This made her a romantic, Brontë-like figure to me, and I admired her even more. I wished that I had such a romantic story.

Unlike most of us in the convalescent ward, Clare spent little time in front of the television – which was still a novelty to us – or gossiping, yet she always seemed to be doing something. She must have written hundreds of letters and received as many answers. When she was not writing she was reading or doing crosswords (she introduced me to solving cryptic clues). In dry weather she went for walks on her own, which made some of the women say she was a snob. She was not – just different from them, with different values and ideas, which I lapped up like a hungry cat with a saucer of milk.

"You should always find something constructive to do with your time, Jean," she would say. "That way you will leave here prepared for your future; otherwise you will have thrown away a big part of your life and you will regret that."

I took her advice, for which I am still grateful, by asking the occupational therapist if I could learn dressmaking. I blush when I think of the first garment I made – a blouse in a horrible sludgy shade of green, which I thought suited my new serious approach to life, with a bow at the neck which never quite sat right. It could not have been admired more if it had been stitched by Christian Dior himself. The only one daring to tell the truth was Mum, who said the colour was too old for me and took all my colour away, but the opinions of my fellow patients were much more important to me.

I had already been taught to type and do Pitman's shorthand by the teacher assigned to tutor me, as I was not yet school-leaving age. How wonderful the welfare system was to me I did not appreciate until I was long back out into the world.

Like all my friends, I soon had to say goodbye to Clare. She came walking up the ward one Friday, after results day, with the tears streaming down her face, contradicted by a grin the width of the Clyde Tunnel. She was being discharged. The drugs had worked for her after a stay of only four months. I really wanted to be happy for her, but my feelings were a mixture of sadness at losing another friend and jealousy that it was not me. It seemed unfair after all the hoops I had been put through that there was no word of my going home. I managed to hide what I felt quite well, signing her good-luck card from the ward and giving her a poem I had written as a farewell present.

She confirmed all my good thoughts of her when she held my hand on the day she was leaving and said, "I know how you must feel, dear, but your turn will come very soon and the time you have spent here is not wasted. I know you are going to start on a wonderful new life very soon," she smiled, "and to tell the truth I'm a wee bit jealous of you. I know lots of people say it, but I mean it. I will keep in touch and I hope you will do the same."

And she did, for a long time. It was I who stopped writing. Friends moved in and out of my life too quickly for me to keep interested in them for very long.

I wonder now about Clare and all the others. I wonder if they remember what a pain in the neck I was – I hope not.

My big day did come a few weeks after Clare left. I was being transferred to Hairmyres Hospital in East Kilbride – for surgery, which Dr Morton assured me would lead to a complete cure.

Ina too had good news. She was going home and her aunt had agreed to give her a home. I did give a fleeting thought to what it would be like for her living with her rapist cousins. I didn't like to ask her and she did not tell me if she had any fears at all. She was just "glad tae be outta here an' back tae a normal life".

So it was goodbye to Law Hospital for good – or so I thought.

CHAPTER 10

MRS GOD BLESS YOU AND OTHER GOOD SOULS

We always heard her before we saw her: "God bless you, m'dears. How are we all tonight?"

Every Friday night, just after tea, she would arrive like a noisy good fairy. She wasn't the size of tuppence, as my mother used to say, but enough energy and goodwill exuded from her little figure to light up 100 Christmas trees. She must have been well into her seventies – even allowing for my adolescent conviction that anyone over twenty was ancient – and she always wore her shiny navy-blue uniform, showing off the whiteness of her huge crown of hair under her Salvation Army bonnet.

She would go around the ward distributing copies of *People's Friend*, *Woman*, *Schoolfriend* and even *The Dandy* and *The Beano* – something for every taste – while asking how we were and delivering messages from their children to the patients whose children were in homes while their mothers were ill. Her visits were indeed a godsend on Friday nights after the X-ray results in the morning, which were not always good for everybody.

I can still remember all of her songs to this day, and one in particular still cheers me up:

It doesn't cost you anything to S, M, I, L, E.
It doesn't cost you anything to S, M, I, L, E.
Throw away your troubles and they'll vanish like the bubbles
If you S, M, I, L, E.

Some of the Roman Catholics refused her magazines and didn't join in her songs, but others did, guiltily.

She always finished off with 'Keep Right on to the End of the Road' and nobody seemed to see the irony of her song choice. For me she was one of the lasting happy memories of that bleak place, overlooked by the blackness of the coal bing.

There were others who gave up their time to visit us, either from the goodness of their hearts or from a sense of duty: the Church of Scotland minister from the local parish church came every couple of weeks. He tried hard to do what I suppose was part of his pastoral role, where we were concerned, but the poor man seemed to be permanently embarrassed when faced with all those attractive-looking women and girls in their beds. He stayed longer at the beds of the long-term patients and the older women – maybe he felt safer with them. When it came to the likes of Flora, who always asked him awkward questions about the Bible, or Ina, who blushed and giggled, or me, who just wished he would go away, the soul was totally inadequate and I'm sure had nightmares about us.

The Catholics were polite and distant with him and he never asked them "to join me in a wee prayer" as he did with the rest of us. They had visitors from their own faith, including an elderly red-faced priest who reminded me of Mr Pickwick. I think he was just as embarrassed as the Protestant minister by this part of his duty, but he hid it better behind the kind of jollity and references to the Holy Father which transferred the embarrassment to us – his captive audience. The Hughes family adored him, and he always seemed to be there when they needed him – when Betty died and then Margaret, the next sister after Mary, who was taken to a Glasgow hospital and did not respond to treatment. Mary told me he was a 'real saint' who visited their home regularly to see that Jimmy and Sally (the one remaining sister) were 'bearing up'.

The other visitors to the Catholic patients fascinated me. They were a group of three nuns. (When I told Dad about them he said Three Nuns was the name of a brand of tobacco. He thought this was very funny, but I was annoyed at him for making fun of them.) I wanted to get to know them. I felt that I would learn something from them – I had no idea what I was looking for, but I made a point of smiling when they passed my bed. They did not visit everyone, only devout Catholics like Margaret Harriday, Jenny Christie and one or two others.

Flora loathed them almost as much as the Church Ladies, saying they were like vampires 'with their big black cloaks'. She told me she'd read a book back home called *The Awful Disclosures of Maria Monk*, which was banned by the Roman Catholics, who burnt every copy they came across. She said it showed how evil nuns were and everyone else to do with the Roman Catholic Church. This only made me all the more determined to somehow get talking to the three nuns – or one of them at least.

It was Sister Taylor of all people who gave me the opportunity. Nurse McKinnon had told her that I was 'top of the class' – my words – in French at school, and on one of her rounds she brought one of the nuns to my bedside.

"This is Sister Boniface," she blushed. "She comes from Paris, you know, and she says you can practise your French on her. Would you like that?"

I felt that every eye in the ward was on me – particularly Flora's – as they all knew I came from a staunch Proddy, Rangers-supporting family.

I heard myself say – and I hoped Flora didn't – "*Oui, Madamoiselle, je cette aime*."

Sister Taylor bridled like a courting pigeon, with pride, and motioned the other sister to take a seat by my bed.

I felt so excited and superior. Surely I was the only person in the ward who could speak to the exotic creature in her own language.

The little snob in me burgeoned into full bloom as she asked "*Comment appelez-vous?*" and I answered "*Je m'appelle Jeanne*," smirking with the knowledge that my name as it is spelt in Scotland would translate as John and using the French version instead.

I had been good at French at school, but I had only been in

the third year when I left, so our conversations were limited to simple exchanges. Still, I enjoyed her visits over the next few weeks because of the superior status if gave me in the ward and with Sister Taylor, who was beginning to believe that she was nursing a child genius. She even began to call me 'Mam'selle' when she gave me my medicine and my mail in the mornings. I had changed my feelings towards her and no longer sniggered cruelly at her shyness in the presence of men and the way her cheeks wobbled when she was angry. I was beginning to grow up and appreciate her obvious good qualities.

Another offshoot of my conversations with Sister Boniface was that I entered a really religious phase that could only be called 'holier than thou' as I talked and wrote boringly about God's purpose and how He would make us all better in His own time, and that we only had to pray and have faith. I bored even myself, and my friends started avoiding me, particularly as I had developed a sanctimonious "Tut-tut!" every time they blasphemed (Ina had a habit of saying "Jeeesus Christ!" when she was the slightest bit annoyed or surprised at anything – which happened a lot) or mentioned sex.

Thank God my holy phase did not last long or they might have killed me, I was so annoying.

The hospital almoner was another regular visitor, particularly to the mothers in the ward. She helped them with keeping in touch with their children's schools and in family-allowance matters. If the children were in care, as some of them were – where the dad had been unable or, in some cases, unwilling to look after them on his own – she kept them in touch with the carers. There was much more she did, and all of the women relied on her visits, but I was still too selfish to be that interested in what she did for others – I was more interested in what she was going to do for me when she first visited me just after my fifteenth birthday.

She told me that as I had reached school-leaving age, but was unable to work, I was entitled to a small allowance from the government, as she put it, of ten shillings and sixpence a week. I was as thrilled as if I was getting my first pay packet and began writing out complex budgets for savings, etc., which I never stuck to. I spent it all most weeks and sometimes I 'lent' it to Eddie and Robert when they visited me.

The most exciting outside visitors kept us in a state of excitement for days before they were due to appear. They were the concert parties. They came about once a month, but sometimes there was a longer gap between visits, as Law Hospital was a bit out of the way for them to travel to more often. Well, that was what I thought, but Ina told me it was because we had TB and a lot of people were scared of catching it from us.

This was probably not completely true, but I believed what Ina told me. I learned later to appreciate what it takes for people to give up their time after work to come and entertain hospital patients in the back of beyond.

It was usually a Monday evening when they came, so we didn't get a film that week. Some people resented that, but most of us loved the live entertainment, particularly – for my pals and me – if there were young men in the party.

From the end of 'rest hour' until teatime we preened and polished ourselves and one another – like women preparing to visit the Sultan in a harem (or so I described it to myself, having just finished a book about a woman being kidnapped and made one of the many wives of an Arabian prince). Ina would wear her tightest T-shirt and give off her familiar aroma overlaid with Evening in Paris, which was her favourite perfume; Big Mary would put on one of the satin blouses she loved, over tight trousers; Flora, in a fluffy cardigan she loved because her dad had bought it and with her hair 'finger-waved' by Nurse McKinnon, looked like a Dutch doll (the two bright-red spots on her pale cheeks looked like too much rouge); and I wore the tartan shirt which my big sister had sent me from London (they were 'the very latest thing', she said in her letter) and the black trousers Mum had bought me. Nurse McKinnon did my hair too.

We were always first in the rec, so that we could sit in the front row and be noticed by any nice-looking fellas in the party. Ina always fell in love with at least one of the performers – usually male, but sometimes she made us blush by saying she fancied 'a go' with some nice young girl singer or dancer. Looking back, the performers were just ordinary people who satisfied their desire to be on the stage while getting a rosy glow from doing good. We saw them as glamorous, desirable stars and even went so far on occasions as to ask for autographs. I blush to think what they must have thought of us, but they filled a need in our lives – the need for glamour and excitement, which other young girls would be getting from going dancing and going out with fellas.

There came a wonderful day, however, when a real singing star visited Law Hospital to entertain us. His name was Dickie Valentine – probably few remember him now, but he was as big a star in those days as any of the present-day pop singers are now. And he was a heart-throb!

The story behind his visit was said to be that his Scots wife's sister had had TB and this was his way of saying thanks for her being cured. I never found out if the story was true or not, but he was our hero for taking the time to sing to us while he was appearing in Glasgow.

He came on a Friday afternoon, as he was performing at night – I think it was in the Glasgow Empire – and even people who didn't go to the usual concerts, bed-patients and on- and off-duty nurses and other staff, crowded into the rec.

He was marvellous. His appearance was quite foreign-looking, Ina said, with his dark curly hair, slightly oriental eyes and sallow complexion. We all agreed that he had the nicest smile we had ever seen. He sang 'The Finger of Suspicion' (I thought Ina would faint) and others I cannot remember now, including some requests from the audience, and chuckled and blushed like a boy when we screamed in ecstasy. He gave out autographed pictures to anyone who wanted them. He really was a star! When I read of his death in a car crash at the age of forty-one, in 1971, I felt that the world was a sadder place.

It was a blessing that we had the good times of the concert parties and Dickie Valentine's visit, because there was a lot of sadness and grief awaiting so many of us.

There were so many people to say goodbye to, knowing we would never see them again.

Part 2

HAIRMYRES HOSPITAL

CHAPTER 1

NEW FRIENDS

Hairmyres Hospital in East Kilbride was the place where patients were sent if they were deemed to require surgery – sometimes after all else had failed – to remove the diseased parts of their lungs. There was a medical ward where we were fattened up for the surgeon's knife. It was like a kind of waiting room between life and death, and the atmosphere was entirely different from that of Law Hospital.

In Law Hospital I had heard it talked about as a place some patients were desperate to go to – seeing it as the next stop before going home cured – but others dreaded it as being their last chance: all the wonder drugs which the wonderful physician Sir John Crofton had proved could cure most cases of TB having failed in their case.

We heard, from patients who had been there or had friends there, that it was entirely different from Law Hospital: "The patients are allowed to smoke if they like, but not in the surgical ward, and they're allowed into the hospital canteen. Some of them even take the bus into East Kilbride. And there are two male wards in the same building! It's great, so it is."

When I listened to all of this, I had not yet been told that there was any possibility that I might have to go there, and I felt a mixture of envy that I was going to miss out on the male wards and a smugness that, according to my X-rays, the drugs were winning the fight for me. Everything pointed to a return to the outside world in the near future, although I had

had a few months of a setback (as Sister referred to it) with the haemorrhage, which Dr Morton said was probably a good thing in the long run. I had no idea what she meant, but as always her word was gospel to me. After a week of bed rest I was allowed time up again and was soon back to going for walks in the grounds or visiting the rec with my visitors. The horror of the liver-like blood clots filling my sputum can was soon fading.

I was moved to Ward 26, which we called the convalescent ward. It was where people generally spent some time before being discharged. It was also a prelude to being transferred to Hairmyres, but I knew that did not apply to me.

Now that Clare and Ina were gone, I felt sure that it was only a matter of weeks before I would hear my own good news.

X-ray results day arrived with the usual dolling-up and excitement. My name was called last – the curse of having a surname beginning with W. Both Dr Ballantine and Dr Morton were there, looking, I thought, particularly pleased with themselves. I was suddenly sure that they were going to tell me I was ready to go home.

"We are very pleased with your progress, Jean." It was Dr Ballantine who spoke, which was a rarity – some said because he stuttered, others that he was just shy with women. He went on, looking at my X-ray, which was on the desk in front of him, rather than at me, "We have arranged for you to see Mr Richards at Hairmyres. Your treatment will be completed there and you will be discharged when that is done."

"What treatment?" I wanted to scream. "What more can be done to me?" But I just sat looking dumbly from one smiling face to the other, like some bewildered tennis spectator.

"It will be much better for your parents too," Dr Morton put in. "Your dad tells me he has managed to get a house in East Kilbride, all ready for you going home. It won't be long now."

"I thought I had had all my treatment," I managed to croak.

They looked at one another and smiled.

"Oh no, dear. You are a hundred times better than you were when you came in . . . very, very ill." Dr Ballantine shook his head. "But it was always realised that to be completely cured you would need surgery. Nothing to worry about – Mr Richards is the best there is. He is a wonderful man. You are very lucky that he has agreed to see you. This is the final lap for you, Jean. Do not let us down now – keep that fighting spirit that has got you this far."

Dr Morton patted me on the shoulder and saw me to the door.

Everyone was excited and glad at my news, except me, and I went along with the party feeling – another two patients were being discharged – not letting on how let down and terrified I felt.

Hairmyres was much more attractive on the outside than Law Hospital. The sanatorium and surgical wards (for TB) looked like an old-style cottage hospital, which it probably had been in its day. A tree-lined avenue led to the building in which I was to spend the next six months of my life. It was three storeys high, painted white, with a sloping slate roof, whereas Law Hospital was a collection of long flat-roofed buildings, which looked not unlike the factory farms which later became blots on the landscape.

For the first few weeks I was put into Ward 2, the all-female TB ward, which was much smaller and more homely than the thirty-bed ward I had become used to. But before being shown to my bed there I had to be seen by the head chest surgeon, Mr Richards, and his colleague, Mr McDonald.

I was a different girl, stepping off the ambulance which took me to Hairmyres, from the poor wee soul who had been trundled down that long corridor at Law Hospital. My hair was now shiny, eyes bright with life, plump cheeks and – miraculously – no cough.

I felt the colour drain from my cheeks when I was taken into the presence of the legendary Mr Richards. He was very tall and heavy-looking – like a huge bear – and his face resembled that of a cod on a slab, with his droopy pale-blue eyes and thick wet lips. There was no kindness in those eyes as he stared at me as if I was something under a slide on a microscope.

The other man spoke first: "Come and sit down here, lass, where we can see you," he said, guiding me towards a seat between where they stood at either side of a huge desk. "I'm Mr McDonald and this is my colleague, Mr Richards. We're going to see that you leave here a fit and healthy young woman."

I was so pleased at being referred to as a young woman that already I knew I would like this man. I looked at him for the first time. He was so different from Mr Richards – it was as if someone had deliberately created two opposite beings. He was small in height – about five foot six – round and jolly, with eyes that twinkled behind NHS glasses which magnified them, giving him what I can only describe as a naughty-boy look.

Mr Richards interrupted him and spoke to the ward sister who had brought me in: "Help the patient to undress, Sister," he rumbled as if he was telling her to perform some unpleasant action.

I unbuttoned my favourite angora top – I had been warned not to wear anything I had to take over my head – and Sister gently slipped down the straps of the lacy-edged vest Mum had bought me. I did not yet have breasts which could fill a brassiere, much to my regret.

"Stand up," he commanded, and I did, folding my arms across my chest. He took my hands down and turned me around, poking and prodding as he did so. "We'll need to see some more meat before anything can be done," he said, and then, giving a noise that maybe passed for a chuckle in his cold world, "You'll have to fatten her up for us, Sister."

He then sat down and started reading a file on the desk. He was finished 'seeing' me.

Mr McDonald had been smiling kindly at me as this went on. He nodded to Sister and she began to help me get dressed.

"You've made great progress, lass. It won't be long now until you're breaking a' the young lads' hearts. Just do what Sister tells you and eat up your food."

He guided me out through the door, giving my elbow a wee squeeze as we went.

That was my introduction to the two men who would be the

most important in my life for the next six months. One would nearly ruin it and the other would save it.

Another man was not completely happy about me being in this much freer place. My dad was glad that I was going to be operated on by the man everyone said was the best, but he was worried that I was going to be allowed to wander in the grounds, go to the café, and mix with some rough-looking women, as he termed them, and, worst of all, men!

The first ward I was in was all-female, then I was transferred to the surgical ward, one end of which was a ward with ten beds, two cubicles, each with four beds for women patients, followed by the duty room. There was the same arrangement at the other end of the corridor, only occupied by male patients. It thrilled me to the marrow to meet with these exotic creatures in the communal corridor as they went to and from their washrooms, which were next to ours, and to meet them in the grounds on our walks. Hairmyres was more than fine by me.

We were even allowed – depending on which sister was on duty – to go along to the men's end in the evenings sometimes to play cards and chat. They taught me how to play Newmarket and five-card brag. They also made me aware that I was attractive to the opposite sex. Mind you, as they were away from their womenfolk – some for a long time – a heifer would probably have been attractive to them. Still, their attention boosted me no end and I flirted like mad. I had just been discovering the excitement of fancying boys and fantasising with my pals about what it would be like to have a boyfriend – winching and all that – when TB had come along and put a stop to all that. Since then my contact with men had been confined to my dad, brothers, hospital porters, doctors, radiologists and my borstal-boy pen pal, so I suppose I was just ripe for making the best of the close contact I had with my new male friends.

I can remember some of their names still, although I never kept serious contact with any of them once I was free.

Andy McCall was a balding man of forty-ish. He was really funny, making suggestive remarks that I didn't always understand and had (I thought) lovely, droopy, sexy eyes.

Jimmie Mason, had a dark Celtic face and a desperate expression. He was an ex-miner, in his twenties, and was always talking about how he 'needed a wumman', which made me go red and giggle with excitement. Once or twice he came into my dreams and I could not look at him the next day.

And Willie Rankin was tall, good-looking, with dark-blonde hair and blue eyes. He was a master at making a young girl think he was in love with her – even though she knew he was married and had two weans. I'm sure if he had got me alone in a quiet place for long enough, he could have done anything with me. He was the only one of my 'boyfriends' who got in touch after I left the hospital, but I did not go to meet him, as he asked. Dad went instead.

I had been home about a month when I got his letter and really I had forgotten all about how I had felt for him. I was becoming wiser and, looking back, I could see through his sly game.

It was a bit like a scene from some Victorian melodrama when Mum put the letter down beside my breakfast one Saturday morning. I opened it as casually as I could, with several pairs of eyes watching me, cursing my fair skin for blushing as soon as I began to read. I cannot remember it word for word as I did not have time to take it all in before Dad took possession of it.

He said that he 'still loved me' and had never stopped dreaming about what we would do together when he 'could get me all to himself at last'. The sentences that followed made tears of anger and embarrassment come to my eyes. They were dirty and horrible to an innocent – as I was, despite my attempts at sophistication – and I wondered how I had appeared to him to make him write to me like that. He finished by saying that I was to meet him that day 'outside the Willow Café. If you're not there I'll come to your house and see your Mum and Dad.'

My cheeks were not red any longer. They were white with panic and fear. I realised that I could not even picture him any longer.

"What's wrong with you?" Mum asked. "Are you sick? You've gone white as a sheet."

Dad looked around his paper. It took a lot to take him away from the racing section on a Saturday morning, but, as always, I was his first priority – even above Peter O'Sullevan, the racing tipster.

"It's a letter from someone in the hospital," I said. Why didn't I say 'some man'? "They want me to meet them today, at the Willow Café."

"That's nice," Mum said. "You met a lot of nice lassies in there. Who is it?"

"It's not a lassie," I said, staring down at the letter. "I'm not going."

I got up from the table and left the room before anything else could be said. All I could think of was him turning up at the house, reminding me how stupid I had been; how he had made me feel by just putting his hand on my neck, or grabbing me around the waist when we met in the corridor. It was as if one of the film stars or characters from novels whom I made up dreams about had come to life. I wanted him to stay where he was in my wee girl's past.

I was sitting on my bed when Dad knocked and came into the room.

"Who is this clown that's writing to you and frightening you like this?" he asked, not unkindly.

"His name's Willie Rankin," I said. "You wouldn't know him. I think he's married."

"Did you let him do anything to you to make him think you would want to meet him?" he asked, and I could see him getting that mad look he got when someone made him angry.

I did what I always did when I thought that I might be in trouble – I started to cry.

"Wheesht," he said, "I'm no angry at you, but a married man has no right getting in touch wi' a young lassie and asking her to meet him. Give me the letter. Don't worry, I'm not going to read it – just make him take it back when I meet him."

I handed him the letter, soaked and crushed as it was, and he stuck it in his trouser pocket.

"Now you go and wash your face and go downstairs. Your

mammy doesn't need to know about this. I'll deal wi' Mr Willie Rankin."

I supposed he had recognised Willie from seeing him around the hospital. All he told me was that he had been 'a bit green about the gills' when he approached him outside the Willow Café and told him never to contact me again or his wife would hear all about it, after he had kicked hell out of him.

So that was the end of my first love affair that never really got started, but it did bring back memories of Ward 2 at Hairmyres Hospital that made me blush for the young fool I had been.

I had never had such close contact with men before – sitting on their beds, playing cards, pretending I could read their fortunes from their hands and lapping up the admiration from those sexually frustrated men, believing that I was as desirable as they made me feel. Looking back I can see that it was a harmless game to them – one they would never have taken any further than flirting and making suggestive pretty-harmless remarks.

Willie was different. He had a darker purpose than the rest. He knew I was a cherry ripe for plucking and he intended to be the one to oblige. At twenty-five he was almost ten years older than me and he had a wife, who visited him three times a week, and two children under five. That was not going to stop him. He came near to making his move sometimes as we walked in the grounds, but there were always other patients around and nurses scurrying to and from the nurses' home. The chance was too dangerous to take. He obviously decided to wait his time until we were both back in the outside world. I can see now that he was grooming me for the day when he could take what he wanted from me. He had not reckoned with the short life of a girlish crush, especially when there were young unmarried men in my life now and Hairmyres seemed years in the past.

"What on earth did ye see in that glaikit-lookin' clown?" Dad asked when he told me there was no need to worry about him contacting me again. "He's far too old for you an' he's got buck teeth like a piano keyboard. I think maybe we should get your eyes tested."

The thing was – although I didn't tell him this – the slightly buck teeth were one of the features that I found attractive about him. They gave his smile a kind of mischievous look, which made me blush, wondering if he was reading my mind. Few people in Scotland in those days had perfectly straight white teeth; at least his were clean and white, with no gaps, unlike the majority of folk, especially in Glasgow.

Dad's question sent me back to my days in Hairmyres. I knew what made Willie attractive to me: he was the first man to touch my neck in a certain way, to wink at me when we were in a crowd as if we shared a great secret, to tell me he wanted to make me squeal and to kiss me on the lips (not as the wee boys at school tried to do, but as a man kisses a woman he is going to make love to). He made an impression on me when I was open to impressions, but he did not leave the lasting memories of others that I met there.

My wee girl's head was turned by the attention the men gave me. They would cheer and shout, "Over here, hen! Come and sit on my bed and we'll talk about the first thing that comes up!"

I had to ask one of the older women what was meant by this, and I don't know who was more embarrassed at the telling – her or me.

"You be careful wi' these men, Jean," she said. "They're missing their wives, and men really need thur hole, ye know. Don't encourage them too much – especially that Willie Rankin and his pal Andy. They would jump on you if they got the chance. Maybe you shouldna go up to the men's end so much. You'll get a bad name about yersel' an' you widnae want that."

She wasn't the only one who noticed my enjoyment of mixing with the men. There was a woman in the ward – a Mrs Hume (good name for her as it turned out) – who was always poking her nose in where she was not wanted. None of the others liked her as she was always moaning and seeing the worst in everything. She'd had more than one patient in tears with her tales of operations that had failed and people who had 'only lasted a year outside'. Apart from her ugly nature, she was ugly to look at, so I avoided her whenever I could. She had a strangely small face dominated by a pointed nose that seemed to have a permanent twitch like a mouse smelling for cheese. This was perched on a long neck above a pear-shaped body dressed in bum-revealing trousers and holey jumpers she knitted herself.

Dad and I had been spending visiting hour in the canteen, laughing over a crossword puzzle. When he got up to leave I noticed her standing just outside the door as if she was waiting to speak to him. I could see him bending slightly to hear what she had to say, his expression changing from polite interest to brow-bristling anger as he turned back to me.

"I need to talk to you," he said, although the bell that told us visiting time was over was already ringing.

I walked with him out of the canteen and saw Mrs Hume making quickly for the entrance to the ward. I had no idea what she could have been saying, but Dad soon put me right.

"What's this about you making a wee hairy o' yersel' wi' a lot of old men?" he snarled at me as we walked back towards the ward.

"What do you mean?" I asked, knowing full well where this poison was coming from. The old bitch! Just when everything was going well! I was getting closer to getting out; the family was happy, because they didn't have to travel so far to visit me at the weekends; I had new friends, who made me laugh and feel good; and now this evil old woman was telling tales on me. My first thought (remembering what had happened with Hetty) was that Dad would have me sent back to Law Hospital, but that was not to be. He was as anxious for me to stay there and get the surgery I needed as I was. Yet he couldn't have me corrupted by a bunch of 'sick, sex-mad clowns'. Something would have to be done. I thought crying might help. It didn't. He insisted on having a word with Sister McLean after he'd made sure I was safely back in the female end of the ward.

The result of this conversation was that I was no longer

allowed to visit the men's end in the evenings, and when I went for a walk in the grounds I had to be accompanied by one of the older women at all times. Mrs Hume volunteered for this duty with a mixture of self-sacrifice and relish. I made a point of never speaking to her on those walks, even when she spoke directly to me.

The new rules did not stop Willie coming along to see me – as long as Sister McLean was off duty – or of joining in the walks in the grounds. Some of the other men came too and we enjoyed baiting my 'jailer' until she was near to tears with rage at times.

I was getting to know the other women in the ward too. My favourite was a girl called Morag McCall, who reminded me a lot of Clare Meichan, who still wrote to me from her home in Largs. She was the only bed-patient in the surgical ward, which seemed odd as we were always being told that we had to be fit and strong to undergo the operations. For example, I was always being nagged to gain more weight before I would even be considered fit for the knife, as one of the nurses colourfully put it. I ate as much as I could of the hospital food, supplemented by loads of food from home, yet I seldom gained an ounce. I began to cheat by putting heavy objects in my dressing-gown pocket on weighing days – paperweights, scissors, small change, anything at all to make that stubborn needle move.

Mr McDonald joked with me about it on his rounds: "Two pounds gained this week, Jean. Keep this up and we'll be calling you 'chubby chops'."

My worry about my weight was nothing compared to those weighing on Morag's fragile, bony shoulders. I noticed that she never lay down, even after lights out. She was propped straight up with the help of a metal grid and about a dozen pillows, and the screens were often around her bed while the nurses attended to her. I wanted to know why, but I was scared to ask. I found out too soon.

I often went to talk to her in the afternoons. She shared my obsession with crosswords and helped me a lot to decipher the more difficult cryptic clues. It was when she leaned forward to take her medication from Sister that I noticed the tube leading from her back – through an opening in her nightgown – to a huge glass bottle at the back of her bed. The bottle was full of something which looked like thick, dirty milk. I felt as if I was going to boak and swallowed as hard as I could, studying the newspaper puzzle as if I had seen nothing. She sat back and let out the saddest sigh I have ever heard.

"Don't worry, pet," she said. "It disgusts everybody, including me. Do you want to leave the puzzle for now?"

I shook my head, although I did want to leave.

"What is it, Morag?" I asked, feeling very stupid.

"I've got emphysema pretty bad," she said. "I have to have a drain in to keep my lungs clear. But don't worry – Mr Richards says I'm getting better."

I couldn't understand then why she laughed when she said this. I did later.

Another patient, Sheila McLean, waiting for a pneumonectomy (the removal of the whole lung), told me Morag's story:

"You should have seen her when she came in here at first," she said. "She was beautiful – like a fashion model. She was allowed up like the rest of us and she was on Mr Richards's waiting list. I think she was content to wait her turn, like everyone else, but her mum and dad wanted to get her fit and out of here as soon as possible – they went private."

I hadn't any idea what she meant.

"They paid Mr Richards to operate on her before her turn. He's got private patients as well as us common people, you know. His private ward is that one just at the top of the driveway – with the nice curtains."

I had seen it, but thought it was just another ward. Apart from the curtains, it looked just like the one we were in.

"What happened?" I asked.

"Oh, she was fine at first," she said. "Well, for a couple of weeks anyway. I've heard that she wasn't making the progress she should – something wrong with the wound – not healing right, or something." Noticing my shock at what she was saying, she tried to reassure me: "Oh, don't worry, pet – it's very rare for anything to go wrong after an operation. I've heard some of the nurses saying it was because she wasn't really ready for it the first time and that's why it happened. She should maybe have waited her turn, eh?"

The spite in her last remark made me want to walk away from her, but I wanted to hear the rest of my friend's story.

"The first time?" I asked.

"Mr Richards said he could put it right with another operation, done right away. Her daddy paid for that one as well."

She sounded spiteful again, and again I ignored it.

"She was out for six months and came back the way you see her now. He says he'll take the whole lung away now – when she's fit for the operation. She'll have to wait this time – her dad can't afford to pay. Anyway, Morag knows that she'll never be fit. She'll never admit it, but she knows."

I walked away then, disgusted and choked with tears. I felt crushed for Morag, but my main feeling was fear for myself. Until then the danger I faced had never presented itself so clearly to me. I had thought of the surgery as just the final step in my recovery – when I had thought about it at all. Now I saw it as an obstacle which I might not overcome. Mr Richards took on the persona of a ruthless butcher in my mind, and I cringed every time he stopped at my bed on his rounds. I even avoided sitting with Morag for a day or two lest she would read what I knew in my face. When I went back to sit by her bed after a couple of days I did not explain why I had stayed away, but I guessed she knew.

The surgical ward was a much more dramatic and emotionally highly charged place than Ward 2, where I had first been taken in Hairmyres. It had a giggly girls'-night-out atmosphere about it. Some of the women there had had their surgery and were just waiting to be discharged; the others – like me – were waiting to be moved to Ward 2. We were all waiting for something, and the feeling reminded me of that daredevil mood I remembered from the last day of school, before the start of the holidays.

My sex education continued there and I had my first experience of being drunk as a monkey.

There were eight of us in what was referred to as the 'big' ward. The other patients occupied smaller side wards as they had other lung problems than TB. Some had bronchiectasis, others diabetes and a few asthma. We did not really see much of them as they stuck to their own small territory.

Madge McNally, a big, loud girl who was the kind of leader of our ward, said of them, "They're scared they might catch the bug off us – silly cows!"

As we had all been told our sputum tests were negative, and therefore we were not contagious, I suppose they were silly for being afraid of contact with us, but who could blame them?

Besides Madge, who was a striking big-busted girl – common as muck, some said – there was Marion Higgins, a quiet girl with a broad, flat face and sallow skin lit up by shiny brown eyes, which always seemed on the verge of tears or laughter.

There were a couple of older (in their thirties) married women, who made little impression on me apart from driving me mad by trying to mother me at every turn. Then there was Edna – not much older than me, but much prettier – just living, like all of us, for the day she would get home. She was having a chaste fling with the paper boy who visited the wards every evening on his round. He was good-looking in a cocky, 'look at me' kind of way. His name was Eddie, and I was jealous that he never even looked my way. They were both from East Kilbride, which was to be my new home town when I got out, and I met them years later, when they were a married couple with two boys.

The others that came and went in Ward 2 I have little memory of as sometimes they only stayed for a night or two before being moved to the surgical department and disappearing out of my life.

Madge, Marion and Edna were my main friends, and it was in their company and with their encouragement that I had my first experience of being drunk. The thought of the night it happened still makes me laugh. I wonder if they remember it and how I nearly gave the show away to the night super – an assistant matron who visited the wards during the night to check that everything was all right – by my drunken friendliness.

It was Madge's idea to get one of the ward maids to bring in the drink. We were all sitting on her bed – she had been reading our horoscopes – when she said, "You know, lasses, I'm really fed up the night. Do you know what ah could go?"

We all thought that she would say something about sex, because she was always saying that she was 'desperate for it'.

"I could just murder a drink," she sighed, "a great big gin an' orange."

"I thought you were going to say 'a man'," Marion laughed, and Edna and I giggled, realising we had all slipped up in our thoughts.

"Aye, ah would like one o' them as well," Madge said, "but as there's no much chance o' that a gin and orange would just hit the spot."

One of the ward maids was called Jessie – a wee Coatbridge woman who was always singing and telling dirty jokes. She was really good to the patients and would shop for them and even deliver messages to men in the male ward fancied by the girls. It was she whom Madge chose to carry out the 'secret mission': she was to smuggle in a bottle of Gordon's gin and a bottle of orange juice and hide them in the washroom for Madge to pick up after visiting time on the Saturday. No one thought of asking visitors to do such a thing as we were all sure that they would disapprove and refuse.

At first they were not keen to include me in the scheme, but what could they do? I had been there at the birth of the idea and it was only fair. I suspected that they thought I might clipe if they excluded me, but no one said so.

There was a hysterical feel about the atmosphere between us from first thing on the Saturday. We could hardly look at one another without giggling, and the rest of the ward, including the nurses, were puzzled and fed up with our madness, which showed itself, apart from the giggling, in snatches of singing and dancing around the ward. It reached its peak when Sadie, the ward maid, put her head round the door and gave Madge the thumbs-up. By that time the visitors were beginning to arrive and most of us were getting ready to go with our folks to the canteen or for a walk. For the first time ever I wished that the time would hurry up and pass. I had never had a drink before, yet I was acting like an alcoholic with withdrawal symptoms – so desperate was I to find out what gin and orange tastes like. The very sound of it seemed sophisticated to me and made me feel on an equal footing with my friends.

At last visiting was over; supper was cleared. People were getting ready to settle down, cleaning teeth, making last visits to the washrooms and putting in curlers. Madge passed my bed carrying her toilet bag and towel.

"Come on, ah'll do your hair for you, Jean," she said, grinning like a clown mask.

I grabbed my things and hurried out with her to the washroom, which was empty apart from Marion and Edna pretending to get ready for bed. Madge slunk into the last cubicle in the row and came out carrying something wrapped in her towel and she had the look of a woman who has found her true love.

"Did you get the glasses?" she asked Edna.

"Sister kept an eye on me when I went into the kitchen," she answered. "I couldn't get them, but I managed to take four cups off the breakfast trolley."

She unveiled the thick off-white hospital mugs as if they had been champagne flutes," which started us off giggling crazily.

Madge revealed the contents of her towel – two bottles. One contained the dilute orange juice which was supplied to patients free of charge, and the other – I hadn't realised it would be in a bottle of beautiful green glass, transparent and shiny, with a black-and-silver label – Gordon's gin!

What pleasure I was introduced to that night! First there was the appeal to my sight, then the sound of the liquid gurgling into the delft mugs – tea never sounded like that – and that smell, like eau de cologne, and finally the taste! It made me cough a bit when the spirit hit my throat, but I loved it. My heart was singing after the first swallow. I only had three refills. The others finished the bottle and then we walked arm in arm back to the ward, with my friends trying to keep me quiet all the way.

We sat around on Madge's bed, exchanging stories – mostly about men – with me listening as I had nothing much to tell in that line. I did mention about my jailbird pen pal, which made them laugh and assure me that he would turn up to visit 'wearing a suit wi' arrows on it'. Madge howled. Finally the night nurse convinced us to go to our own beds before the night super came on her rounds.

"It's Hathaway," she said. "You know what she's like. She'll have an Annie Rooney if there's anybody still up. Go on now – it's long after lights out."

The others got into their own beds and lay down obediently, but I couldn't accept that the wonderful night was at an end. I decided (or the gin did) that I would sing a few songs. My favourite at that time was 'Here in My Heart', and I put all my drunken emotion into it. The other patients' shushing was nearly as loud as my singing as they could hear the heavy tread of Hathaway approaching the ward, but nothing could shut me up. I sung on happily, with tears rolling down my cheeks.

The door opened and the night sister hurried in, saying, "What is all this? Is someone having a bad dream?" (So much for my singing!)

Behind her was Assistant Matron Hathaway, shining the flashlight she carried on her rounds. I had just finished the chorus and was taking a deep breath ready for my next song when she came to my bedside. All I could see of her, behind the torch's beam, was her huge white headdress, like the one Sister Taylor, in Law Hospital, had worn, and I came over all homesick for Ward 28.

There was not another sound in the ward (they must all have been holding their breaths) as I said with a sob, "You look just like Sister Taylor. I really miss her, you know. Do you know her? She's the best ward sister in the world." And then, for some reason: "I like you too, but you could never be as nice as her. I love her."

"Come on now," she said, "you're disturbing the other patients. Let Sister and me make you nice and cosy."

Somewhere in the ward someone tittered. She leaned over to straighten my pillows and got a whiff of my ginny breath.

"Sister," she hissed, "this child has been drinking! What on earth is going on here?"

Sister leaned over me and sniffed, nipping my arm hard as she did so.

"There's no way drink could be brought into the ward, Matron," she answered. "It's probably these horrible sweets she's always sucking. They make her breath smell like perfume."

I've always wished I could be as quick-thinking and plausible as she was that night – or was it just that Miss Hathaway was easily fooled? Anyway, they tucked me into my blanket straitjacket and went off to finish their rounds.

Next day the others swore that they would not even tell me when/if they planned another drinking session. It didn't matter, because I was transferred to the surgical ward next day.

CHAPTER 2

A LIFE-SAVING OPERATION

Apart from the male patients and Morag, I didn't get very close to anyone in Ward 2. It was as if most of them had already moved on to their lives outside the hospital. They were so near to being free and going back to family and friends that they did not have the same need to start up friendships as the patients in Law Hospital had had. I became closer and closer to Morag as the weeks of waiting passed, especially when I was barred from visiting my men friends in the evenings. Members of her family often came to speak to me when they were visiting and I was in the ward, particularly her father, the headmaster. His interest in me appealed to my snobbish side. He was just how I pictured a headmaster should look: tall, slightly stooped, with piercing eyes behind gold-rimmed specs, a strong but quiet voice with a proper accent (not put on or pan-loaf) and wearing a tweed jacket with leather patches on the elbows. Later, when I became a teacher, I always hoped to see this ideal in real life, but I never did.

Sometimes the nurses had to attend to Morag while he was visiting, and he would come and talk to me while the mysterious goings-on happened behind the screens. I was proud that he seemed to like to talk to me and asked him about what it was like to be a teacher and if he had to belt pupils sometimes and what you had to do to become a teacher. He always answered me patiently, explaining the ins and outs of being a teacher (I decided then that that's what I would be if

I couldn't be an actress – my first choice) and how he hated hitting people, but sometimes it was necessary to maintain discipline.

His advice about what you had to do was the same thing Dad was always saying to me: "Stick in, work hard and get good qualifications."

He would ask me about my life before I came into hospital, what books I read and what I would do when I got out. He asked me once if it was OK for him to draw me as it was a hobby of his to do charcoal sketches of people 'with interesting faces'. Morag told me that he said I reminded him of Bambi in the Walt Disney film, and I looked at myself in the mirror even more than usual to see if I could see the likeness. I couldn't, but when he presented the drawing to me a few days later he had portrayed me as a wide-eyed fawn – an image I cultivated for a few weeks, much to the consternation of the nurses and my chaperone, Mrs Hume, who thought I was either making a fool of her or making eyes at the men we met on our walks.

I was used to short-lived friendships by now and could usually just shrug off the departure of those I had become fond of; however, Morag's leaving took the heart from me for a while, not just because of the sadness of her going, but because I was losing contact with her father as well.

What made it harder was that I did not even see her go or get to say goodbye. It was a Saturday and my two brothers were visiting me. We went to the canteen, where we had a hilarious time playing our game of people-watching, which involved making up stories about people around us, getting more far-fetched and ridiculous as the game progressed. I was in a funny 'up and down' state when I got back to the ward. I had enjoyed myself and the silly game had really given me a lift, but the downside was that I wanted more than ever to be like them and walk out of this place. I could feel that familiar black cloud coming down on my head as I took off my shoes and lay on top of the covers on my bed. The screens were around Morag's bed. I thought the nurses must be attending to her.

I was lost in reading the serial in *Woman's Own*. Looking over half an hour later, I saw that the screens were still there and there did not seem to be anything moving behind them. I got up and started to walk across to Morag's bed.

"She's no there, pet," one of the older women called. "They took her away at visiting time. She'll be better off at home, poor lass."

The black cloud came down completely; I burst into tears so violent that one of the women went to get the duty nurse. She gently led me back to my bed, where I lay down and covered my head. I just kept thinking over and over, 'Poor Morag, she was so nice! And her poor, poor Dad! Despite all the sad exits I had seen before – the friends I had lost and the stories I had heard – Morag's leaving made me realise how sad, cruel and unfair life can be. I had lost the shell of self-centredness of childhood. It was the first painful truth that had got through to me as a grown-up person, and it almost broke my heart. I thought of how I had been told over and over again that if you kept your spirits up and did not lose heart you would beat the disease and go back to a normal life. It is a lie! Morag had an abundance of fighting spirit, yet the disease still won in the end.

I got a letter from her father telling me that she had 'died peacefully' a few weeks after she had left the hospital. He enclosed a photo of her taken when she was unravaged by disease. I slept with it under my pillow for a long time afterwards. The nurses worried that I was so sad and allowed Wille Rennie and some of the others to visit in the evenings to play cards – much to Mrs Hume's disgust.

It was Mr Richards who chased all thoughts of Morag from my mind by giving me the news that I had been waiting for. It was a Friday morning and he was on his rounds, with only Sister Wilson in attendance; often he was accompanied by other doctors, to whom he showed off as they obviously hung on his every word and laughed at his cruel attempts at humour. This morning he had no audience and seemed to be in a great hurry to get the round over with. Under the white coat could be seen tweed plus fours, so he was probably heading for the golf course.

I know how a baby feels looking up from a cot or pram at the giants looking down on it. That's how I felt every time Mr Richards stopped at the end of my bed and picked up my chart – very small and powerless.

He stared at the chart, muttering to himself, and then threw it on to the bed, stared at me for a full two minutes, turned to Sister and said, "I'll operate on this one on Monday," before shambling out of the ward like a great walrus over rocks.

Everyone was silent at first and then Marion Higgins called over to me, "That's great, hen. You'll be outta here in no time. You'll need to phone home and tell them the good news, eh?"

Voices from all around the ward congratulated me on my good fortune. Nurses, Sister and ward maids all appeared to say how happy they were for me. I was shaking and didn't know what to say to them. Of course it was good news, but I wished it had been anyone but Mr Richards who was to operate on me. I had never got over my fear of him from our first meeting, and what I had heard about his treatment of Morag and other patients filled my mind, instead of the thought of soon being 'cured' and ready to go home.

Marion and Mrs Hume walked me to the public phone at the top of the avenue and I dialled my brother's work, as Dad had told me to do.

It was Robert who came on to speak to me. He seemed a bit puzzled as to why I was phoning – after all, Dad would be visiting me on the Saturday as usual. He did not treat the news as being as shattering and wonderful as it appeared to be to me and the other women then. He was sixteen and the main things in his life were Glasgow Rangers, dancing and the girls in the typing pool.

"Remember to tell Dad," I said. "He said I was to phone right away if there was any word of the operation."

"OK, I'll tell him," he said with a bored sigh. "I have to go. The boss doesn't like us taking calls. Bye."

I was waiting for them, as usual, on the seat at the top

of the drive when they came to visit on the Saturday. Mum was loaded with parcels as if it was my birthday. Dad put his hands on my cheeks and kissed me – much to Mum's and my embarrassment.

"You'll be outta here in no time, hen. We're goin' to do up your room right away." His smile disappeared and his brows met above his nose. "I would have been here last night if that clown o' a brother of yours hadnae forgot to tell me your news until he was goin' to his bed." The smile came back as he put his arm round my shoulders. "Still, never mind that now. Let's go and have a cuppa so's we can talk about you coming out. Your mother'll take your parcels up to the ward for you and meet us in the canteen."

With that we walked away, leaving Mum, like some native bearer, to follow behind when she had delivered the bundles.

When the visitors had left and everyone had seen my presents – a new dressing gown, trousers, sweaters, a skirt and underwear – and gasped over them, we had another visitor to the ward, who changed the mood pretty drastically.

Mr McDonald often made a quick round of the wards on a Saturday evening. Willie Rankin was sitting on my bed, making eyes at me and stroking my neck, when one of the nurses came rushing in and told him to get back to his own ward.

"Mr McDonald is on his way up the stairs," she said. "Shift yourself, quick."

He came bustling into the ward along with Sister Wilson – who was said to be in love with him – and was greeted all round by smiles and hellos. Nobody ever smiled when Mr Richards came in, or said hello. He stopped at the end of my bed and gave me his usual wink.

"Well, how's our cheeky monkey today?" he asked.

I was about to give back a cheeky answer, but Sister interrupted: "Oh, Jean's on top of the world today, Mr McDonald," she simpered. "Mr Richards has put her on his list for Monday. What do you say to that?"

It was the first time I saw him looking other than pleased with the world.

"For what?" he asked, making Sister jump as if she was guilty of something.

"He said a thoracoplasty," she answered.

"No, definitely not," he said. "That's not right." And then, turning back to me and smiling: "Don't you worry, monkey – Sister and I will sort this out. I'll see you on Monday morning – early."

He hurried out of the ward, Sister following on in the half-run, half-walk peculiar to nurses.

As patients we understood almost as much of the technical language as the surgeons and doctors. Mr Richards specialised in the thoracoplasty operation, which as far as we knew meant crushing – or permanently collapsing – the infected part of the lung so that, in theory, the diseased part just died off, leaving the rest of the lung healthy. It meant removing several ribs and often the patients were left kind of lopsided afterwards. 'Better than being dead' was the consensus at Hairmyres.

Luckily I did not have to tell Dad that the operation might be in doubt for Monday as it was the boys who visited on the Sunday and they just wanted to talk about how much they hated staying in the new town of East Kilbride, the latest exploits of Glasgow Rangers and the dancing on the previous night. The operation didn't seem all that interesting to them – just something that had to be done before I was allowed home.

The ward staff and the other patients did not even mention Mr McDonald's visit. They were as confused as I was.

On Monday morning the breakfast was just being cleared away when my hero – as I thought of Mr McDonald – arrived. Sister looked very nervous as they stopped at my bed.

"Now, young lady," he grinned, "you're going to have a little treat this morning. I've had a word with Mr Richards and we've decided to postpone your operation. Oh, don't worry – it won't be for long. Sister will get a nurse to bring you downstairs to see me in the X-ray department as soon as you are ready. Then you will have a very interesting morning."

I was not sure how to respond to his quiet laughter as he hurried on his way.

What followed, when a nurse took me along to see him, was almost as funny as my drunken singing, although it was not meant to be.

I was shown into a consulting room, where, under Mr McDonald's instructions, another nurse inserted a tube down my throat, telling me to swallow and not to boak. He told me to sit down and lean over to the left side while keeping my head still and facing the front.

He then began injecting a thick white liquid into the tube, all the time saying, "Keep over, keep over."

That was when I began to feel like laughing, but I knew if I did I would ruin whatever the treatment was, so I closed my eyes and tried not to think of how ridiculous I must look. Worse was to come!

"Right now, lass," he said, "I want you to stand up slowly and keep leaning to the left. Nurse and I are going to walk you along the corridor to be X-rayed. You're a wee soldier. It'll soon be over."

There was a row of seats on one side of the corridor for patients waiting for X-rays – my bad angel had made sure that they would be fully occupied that day as we walked along. Mr McDonald and a red-faced nurse were at either side of me as I limped comically, listing very much to the left, like a boat about to capsize or Quasimodo without his hump. They kept their eyes straight ahead. I had to look upwards as if pleading for alms. The patients had the decency and self-control not to laugh out loud, as I'm sure I would have done if I had been witnessing our gruesome threesome. It was only really a few yards to the X-ray room, but it was probably the longest walk of my life. However, the outcome was worth it.

After I had been X-rayed from various angles, he showed me the finished films and explained why he had not wanted Mr Richards to carry out his thoracoplasty.

"You see this black mark here, lass?"

He was the most serious I had ever seen him and I nodded, convinced that he was going to tell me something awful – and he did, in a way.

"That's a hole the size of half a crown in your left lung. The only way to deal with it – because it won't ever heal – is to cut out that part of your lung and get rid of the TB completely. I'll make sure that you leave here a strong, healthy young lady."

He took the trouble to explain to me the difference between a thoracoplasty – which Mr Richards had been intending to carry out – and a lobectomy, which he would do instead. It was very technical, but I got the gist and felt very adult about being given the information. No one had ever explained so fully what was happening inside me or shown me films of the damage to my lungs. It was terrifying, yet it made me feel confident that he would make sure that I was going to be all right. I think I was in love with him.

Willie Rankin, Jim and Andy all came to see me the night before the operation and I flirted madly with them. I felt as if I was about to take off into the air above my bed with excitement. Mostly, patients became very quiet on the eve of their operation, but I couldn't wait for it all to begin. I wasn't scared. The feeling was more like being on a ride at the carnival – where we used to go every Christmas – as if my eyes were popping out of my head and I could not stop laughing and talking. The night sister eventually chased the 'boys' back to their own end and told me to lie down and try to get a good night's sleep. How could I, at the start of this adventure with my new hero? I did, eventually, and had to be wakened to go for my pre-op preparations. I got no breakfast and for the first time in my life felt hungry first thing in the morning.

Looking back, I can understand why my behaviour was so different from that of the others. It was my age. Every young person thinks that they are immortal. Whereas the others had the dread of 'something going wrong' – dying under the anaesthetic or, even worse, waking up as they were being cut open – I had no such fears. I was glorying in the drama and being the centre of attention, and behind it all was the knowledge that I was getting nearer to freedom at last.

Even the preparations for the operation interested and excited me, but there was one hitch that nearly panicked me.

A beautiful Indian lady doctor was given the job of inserting a tube into a vein in my ankle, for the drip (there was a problem of getting a suitable vein elsewhere in my skinny body). I was gazing up at the light, totally relaxed, when I felt the worst pain I had ever experienced – it was as if someone was cutting into my flesh, which was actually what was happening. She had cut open the insertion point while I was fully conscious.

"Stop!" I heard Mr McDonald saying. "We'll have to put her under quick – leave that just now." He leaned over me and smiled. "Right, lass, I'm going to give you a little injection now to put you to sleep. You'll soon be back in the ward. Now you can help me by counting backwards from twenty."

I do not know how far I got. The next thing I knew I was back in the side ward and the screens were around my bed. What had happened? What about the operation?

I called weakly for a nurse.

"You're awake," the sister said. "Well, that was no bother to you, was it? Let's sit you up a bit and make you more comfortable."

She and the Nurse gently sat me up so that I could look around. All I could see were the hated beige screens and numerous apparatuses which seemed to be attached to my body.

"Did I not have the operation?" I asked, making them both laugh and shake their heads at one another.

"Of course you did, and it was a great success," Sister answered. "Now all you have to do is have a good sleep until Mr McDonald sees you later. Your mum and dad phoned. They'll be along to see you tonight for a wee while."

It was not long before the pain started and I believed that I really had undergone surgery.

Everybody was amazed and delighted by my quick recovery from what was in fact a revolutionary major operation. Mr McDonald told me that he was not surprised at all.

"You're a wee fighter," he told me. "Before long you'll be waving to us all as you walk down that avenue. Pity help the poor lads in the outside world! You'll create havoc."

I believed him, until one night, after supper, we post-op patients decided to look at our wounds in the mirror. This was almost a ritual – to compare numbers of stitches and whether they were beginning to fade already. It was done by the patient holding up a mirror while another held up a mirror at her back so that the scar could be plainly seen. The other three women were quite happy with theirs – even proud – but I was horrified by what I saw: my left shoulder blade had disappeared; I had been turned into a deformed hunchback. I threw the mirror down and howled so loudly that Sister Wilson came running into the ward. She tried everything to comfort me, telling me that the operation had cured me and soon I would 'build up muscle' and look just the same as everyone else. I didn't believe her and yelled, like a spoiled wee girl, that I was going to run away if she didn't get Mr McDonald to come and see me.

It was just before lights out and I was still making a fuss and upsetting the whole ward despite the soothing words of the nurse whom Sister had told to stay by my bedside, when she walked in accompanied by the man who had been my hero until I had seen what he had done to me.

He came and stood at my left side and ran his hand down where my shoulder blade had been. Sister was staring at him with a really strange look in her eyes, as if she was warning him about something. She shook her head angrily at him as he lifted up my arm, and after a few seconds he put it down again.

"Right, lass," he said, "tomorrow morning I'll see you in the theatre and we'll make you as beautiful as ever. It'll only take minutes and you'll be able to wear a backless gown like any film star. Now I'm off for my supper, which you interrupted."

He was laughing as they left the ward and Sister gave him a little shove, which made me wonder if she fancied him, as the ward gossip had it.

The story was that they had been in love for years, but because of their elderly parents, who needed looking after, they could not marry. It was probably just another romance that lovesick women, as we were, had to make up to keep us happy.

Next morning, under a local anaesthetic, he reset the shoulder, which was dislocated because of the previous surgery, and I returned to the ward with tape round my chest to keep it in place 'until it settles in', as Sister told me. She also told me what her angry look had been about. He had been about to manipulate it back into place as he stood at my bed, but she was not about to let him cause me such pain – even though it would have been over very quickly.

He was still my hero – even when he removed the sticky tape from across my poor wee nipples a week later.

I was happy, in the following weeks, as my strength returned. Mum and Dad spoiled me by bringing all kinds of goodies to tempt my appetite; Willie Rankin, Andy and Jim visited me when they got the chance, flirting and telling me jokes – some of which I didn't understand. One of the jokes was about women without men using a candle for sex. I kind of understood, but pretended not to. Maybe that was why someone sent me a parcel containing a fat, white tallow candle and an obscene poem, explaining how it should be used. I was really hurt by this 'joke', feeling that they were making a fool of me, and refused to speak to the men the next time they visited me. All of them denied it, except Willie, who said I should grow up and learn to take a joke. I enjoyed their attention too much to fall out with them for long, so soon we were back on the old footing.

I had been allowed out for short walks in the grounds for about a week (accompanied by Mrs Hume) when Sister told me that Mr McDonald wanted to see me in the duty room the following morning.

"This means you'll be getting out," Willie said. "I'll not be long after you and we can meet up, without your bodyguard."

He stroked the back of my neck as he said this and I shivered for the rest of the night when I thought about it.

But it was not to tell me I was going home. Mr McDonald was very serious-looking, like a headmaster about to give a severe telling-off, and Sister looked a bit flustered and pink about the cheeks. He did not even wink at me as I sat down in front of the desk.

'The operation didn't work!' was my first thought. 'I am not going home after all.'

"Your dad's been in to see us, Jean," he said. "He's not a happy man."

Mrs Hume had been busy. Apparently she had made a point of meeting Dad when he left at visiting time and told him of the men's visits to me and even about the candle incident.

The result was, as Mr McDonald explained sadly, "You're due to be discharged in three to four weeks, but your dad does not want you staying here any longer. He is convinced that we cannot look after you."

I thought he was going to say that I was being discharged early, but no.

"I'm afraid we'll have to send you back to Law Hospital and you'll be discharged from there," he said, adding, as he saw that I was upset, "Don't worry, lass – you know a lot of people there and I'm sure Dr Morton and Dr Ballantine will be delighted to see you. You're one of their greatest successes, you know, and they deserve most of the credit for your recovery."

I didn't care about any of that. The thought of going back to that dreich place horrified me, and not for the first time I hated my dad and, even more so, Mrs Hume.

Two days later I was taken back to Law Hospital, depression as black as the looming coal bing crushing my happiness. I felt hurt that Mr McDonald had not come to the ward to say goodbye. The next time I saw his name was in a newspaper – thirty-odd years later – reporting his retirement, and I realised that I had never thanked him for saving my life. All I had thought about was my own disappointment at having my freedom curtailed by being sent back to Law Hospital, where I never thanked Dr Morton and Dr Ballantine either. I wasn't abnormally selfish – just young.

Law Hospital was not as bad as I had thought. I was back in

Ward 28 with the same nurses and ward maids, who welcomed me as if I had undergone an ordeal and only they could look after me properly – as they had done for nearly four years of my life. There was no fatted calf, but they had ordered in their version of it for my first night back – fish and chips – and we all sat around two tables pushed together and had a party. I made them all laugh at my descriptions of people in Hairmyres – particularly Mr Richards and my 'bodyguard', Mrs Hume. Even nurses and maids who were off duty came in especially to see me, and seeing them all – including Sister Taylor, Nurse McKinnon, Nurse Brown and Ellen, my favourite ward maid – made me cry like a baby, for I knew I would be leaving all of them behind for good very soon.

Sister Taylor couldn't stop beaming at me when she did her rounds, and the doctors both beamed on me as if I had achieved something to make them very proud. I preened and postured, not realising that the great achievement was theirs and how lucky I was to have been the recipient not only of their medical knowledge, but also of their nurturing and love over the years.

I had been back only two weeks when Friday results day arrived. I had finished the final course of drugs and been X-rayed the previous week; now I waited nervously with the others to be called to the duty room. I knew that the news would be good, but I was scared nevertheless.

I didn't join in the jokes and speculations of the other patients who were waiting to be called. I was the schoolgirl who had been promoted to a higher class and didn't want to play with her old pals any more. I had nothing in common with them. In fact, for some reason I despised their fears and half-hearted jokes. After all, I was cured now. I was not part of the same world as them. That's how much of a pain I was!

"Come away in, Jean!"

I had never seen Dr Ballantine looking so alive and happy. He did not look like Groucho Marx any more. He was quite good-looking really.

“Sit down here.” Dr Morton patted the chair beside her rather than the ‘patient’s chair’ opposite them. “I bet you thought this day would never come. You’re going home, my dear.”

I could only get one word out: “When?”

“As soon as your dad can come for you,” she answered. “Probably tomorrow.”

After a few minutes of smiling, beaming, handshaking and even a hug from Dr Morton, they sent me back to the ward and called in the next patient.

I did the ritual bed tour on the day I was leaving, cards and presents being exchanged and everybody wishing me “All the best, hen.” The suggestive remarks included “Don’t do anythin’ I wouldn’t do” and (one that made Dad’s eyebrows bristle with anger) “Haud on tae yer haepenny!” I had an idea what it meant, and it made me blush because it was said in front of him, but nothing could really put a damper on that day for me – not even when Dad gave me a row for laughing when the young bus conductor flirted with me.

Somewhere a little voice may have warned me that I was not going to be as free as I had imagined in the outside world. There might still be bonds that had to be broken, but for the moment I felt as free as a bird being let out of a cage.